Clinical Leadership
Development

Clinical Leadership Development

A book of readings

Edited by

John Edmonstone

Kingsham

First published in 2005
by Kingsham Press

Oldbury Complex
Marsh Lane
Easthampnett
Chichester, West Sussex
PO18 OJW
United Kingdom

© 2005, John Edmonstone

Typeset in AGaramond

Printed and bound by
Antony Rowe Ltd
Chippenham
Wiltshire
United Kingdom

ISBN: 1-904235-29-8 [paperback]   .
      1-904235-30-1 [hardback]

British Library Cataloging in Publication Data
A catalogue record of this book is available from the British Library

Edmonstone, John

About the editor

John Edmonstone is a leadership, management and organisation development consultant who works in the NHS, local and central government. He has held a range of line, project and human resource management positions and for the last 18 years has run a successful consultancy based in Ripon, North Yorkshire. He is also Senior Research Fellow at the Centre for Health Planning & Management, University of Keele and Associate, Centre for the Development of Healthcare Policy and Practice, University of Leeds. He has been involved in clinical leadership development programmes since 1999.

Contributors

Jay Bevington MA (Hons), DClinPsych is Associate Director of the NHS Clinical Governance Support Team, NHS Modernisation Agency

Collette Clifford MSc, PhD, RGN, DipN, DANS, RNT, ITLM is Professor in Nursing and Head of Research at the School of Health Sciences, University of Birmingham

Mike Cook EdD, MSc (Quality Management), MSc (Education Management), RN, Cert.Ed, Dip.N, ILTM is Associate Dean (Campus Education), St Bartholomew School of Nursing & Midwifery, City University, London

Wendy Cowie MSc, DMS, SRN is an Organisation Development Consultant

Jenny Cowpe BA, MBA, PGCE, MIHM is Senior Fellow, Clinical Management Unit, Centre for Health Planning & Management, University of Keele

Geraldine Cunningham BSc (Hons), RN, Dip.N is Director of the RCN Clinical Leadership Programme at the Royal College of Nursing

Linda Dack BSc (Hons), MSc, RGN, RM, RHV is Development Lead (Allied Health Professionals), Salford Royal Hospitals NHS Trust and LEO Facilitator for the National AHP Leadership Programme

Lesley Downes BSc (Hons), Dip HE, RGN is Assistant Director of Nursing, University Hospital of North Staffordshire NHS Trust

John Edmonstone MSc, is Director of MTDS Consultancy, Senior Research Fellow at the Centre for Health Planning and Management, University of Keele and Associate at the Centre for the Development of Health Care Policy and Practice, University of Leeds

Prof. Christina Edwards MBA, RGN, RHV, MIHM is Director of Nursing with County Durham and Tees Valley Strategic Health Authority and Visiting Fellow, Centre for Leadership and Management, University of York

Ann Foreman DipN, DMS, SRN is Head of Organisation Development for Northumbria Healthcare NHS Trust and Northumberland Care Trust

Jan Freer MSc, MCSP, MACP is Head of Organisation Development, Calderdale & Huddersfield NHS Trust, Honorary Visiting Fellow, Revans Institute for Action Learning & Research, University of Salford and Associate, Centre for the Development of Healthcare Policy & Practice, University of Leeds

Helen Green BSc (Hons), MEd, DMS, RGN, Cert Ed is Assistant Director of Nursing, University Hospital of North Staffordshire NHS Trust

Maggie Griffiths BSc(Hons), MSocSci, RGN is Lecturer/Portfolio Worker at the School of Health Sciences, University of Birmingham

Denise Houghton BA, MBA, RGN, RM, RHV was Director of Nursing, Pennine Acute Hospitals NHS Trust

Sue Inglis MSc (HealthProfEd), PGDipEd, DipMgt, RGN, RM is Head of Learning & External Consultancy, The Learning Alliance

Helen Jones is an independent consultant and Senior Visiting Fellow at the Centre for Leadership & Management, University of York, where she acts as Director of the MA/Postgraduate Diploma programme in Leading Innovation and Change

Jennifer King is Managing Director of the Edgecumbe Consulting Group Ltd, Bristol

Hazel Mackenzie BSc, MSc, RN, RSCN, NCDN, PGCE is the Head of RCN Clinical Leadership , Royal College of Nursing, Scotland

Sophia Martin BSc, MA, M Phil, is an independent development consultant

Nick Nicholson BA (Hons), Dip HSM, Cert. Training is Co-Director, Centre for Leadership and Management, University of York

Calum Paton MA (Oxon), MPP (Harvard), D.Phil (Oxon) is Professor of Health Policy and Director-Designate of the Centre for Health Planning and Management, University of Keele and Chair of the University Hospital of North Staffordshire NHS Trust

Sheila Peskett is a member of the Medical Directors Panel, Centre for Health Planning & Management, University of Keele, for the NHS Leadership Centre's Medical Leadership Development Programmes

Alan Phillips BSc, MA (Management Learning), is a partner in a specialist coaching consultancy and an Associate of the Centre for Leadership and Management, University of York

Karen Picking BA (Hons), MIPD is an Organisation Development consultant

Julia Pokora BSc, MSc, Dip. Counselling is a partner in a specialist coaching consultancy, Coaching For Change, and is Visiting Senior Lecturer at the Centre for Leadership and Management, University of York

Andrew Scowcroft MA, MHSM, MCIPD, FISM, AIMC is Principal, the Development Consultancy, South Wales

Sue Smith BSc (Hons), MBA, RGN, RM, RHV, FWT is Programme Director, Centre for Health Care Policy & Practice, University of Leeds

Amanda Thomas MBBS, DCH, MMedSci, MA, FRCPCH is Consultant Community Paediatrician and Associate Medical Director, East Leeds Primary Care Trust

Julie Werrett BSc is Research Fellow at the School of Health Sciences, University of Birmingham

David Whitney is Professor and Head of the Clinical Management Unit, Centre for Health Planning & Management, University of Keele

David Wilson is an independent consultant based in Harrogate

Fran Woodard MBA, MCSP is National Lead for Allied Health Professionals and Healthcare Clinical Scientists Leadership and Critical Care Programmes, Leadership Centre, NHS Modernisation Agency

Tim van Zwanenberg MA, EdD, FRGP is Professor of Postgraduate General Practice and Director of Postgraduate General Practice Education, Postgraduate Institute for Medicine and Dentistry, University of Newcastle

Acknowledgements

This book has been stimulated by my continuing work as a programme tutor on the national Medical Leadership development programmes run through the Centre for Health Planning & Management at the University of Keele, together with three years part-time working with the Centre for the Development of Healthcare Policy & Practice at the University of Leeds. The experience of working with colleagues in these settings, together with my own consultancy work, has convinced me of the centrality of clinical leadership to the success of health care organisations – and therefore also of the need to develop that leadership. While aware that much excellent work was going on, it was also clear that this emerging good practice needed to be brought together into a single publication which captured the innovation and challenge in as comprehensive a way as possible.

Many thanks are due to all the contributors to this book, every one of whom has been "leaned-on" in various ways to meet deadlines and produce drafts. Thanks are also due to those who were asked or offered, but ultimately were too busy doing clinical leadership development to be able to find the time and space to reflect and write about it.

My thanks are also due to my son, Duncan, for his IT help at a crucial time in this book's production; to my daughter, Rachel, (again!) and son-in-law, Charles, for their word-processing expertise, and finally, to my wife, Carol, who is always supportive when it is most needed.

Who should read this book?

This book is for leaders at all levels in the NHS, spanning board and executive levels to directorate, network and front line leadership roles. It is also of value to those involved in leadership development, education and research.

Contents

Introduction

The original stimulus for this book came on a day when I attended a conference in the very early days of the NHS Workforce Development Confederations. A newly-appointed Chief Executive of a WDC (who shall be nameless, for reasons which will soon become apparent!) delivered a presentation on the new organisation's work programme. A question from the audience asked "Would leadership development feature at all on the WDC's agenda?" The Chief Executive replied in the affirmative, but when asked for some practical examples of this he mentioned only two – the graduate entrant Management Training Scheme (which in various forms has existed within the NHS from the 1950s) and the importance of identifying and fast-tracking potential future NHS managers.

Only a day or so before the then Secretary of State had also been speaking at another conference about the importance of clinical leadership and the significant investment which was then being made in the Royal College of Nursing Clinical Leadership and Leading an Empowered Organisation (LEO) programmes. I was struck powerfully by the way in which the WDC Chief Executive thought and spoke about *management and managers*, while the focus was quite clearly changing to one of *clinical leadership and leaders*.

This gap is, of course, nothing new. Based upon Donald Schon's original work, there has been a useful distinction made between so-called "technical-rational" and "professional-artistry" views of clinical professional practice (Fish & Coles, 1998), while the divide between NHS operational management on the one hand, and practice development for clinical professionals on the other, has also been well highlighted (Page, 1998).

This concern for management and managers can be traced back as far as the 1960s and 1970s, when (stimulated by the new nursing management roles created by the Salmon Report) major investment began to be made in the training of NHS managers. The 1980s saw a further quickening of pace and a widening of focus as the NHS Training Authority's "Better Management, Better Health" report turned attention towards management *development,* rather than simply training. The 1990s and the advent of the internal market in health care placed great emphasis on spotting and developing managerial talent through assessment and development centre methodologies and associated development programmes, but it was probably not until the advent of "Third Way" thinking that the importance of leadership came to be recognised.

What all these earlier approaches seem to have had in common (particularly in the heyday of general management and the internal market) was that they embodied *unitary* assumptions (typically imported from the private sector) that there should be a single belief system and a single power system – that is, management – in health care organisations. Earlier approaches had assumed a more pluralistic and diverse system of contrasting beliefs and power-sources (Edmonstone, 1986) and the latter-day "opening to leadership" seemed to reflect a return to pluralism (Darwin *et al.*, 2002, Attwood *et al.*, 2003).

I have been lucky enough to have bridged the divide between managers and clinical professionals on a number of occasions. My earlier career involved management training for NHS managers; widened-out into management development, before taking a more corporate view with organisation development. More recently I have become very involved in the development of both clinical and managerial leaders, from both academic and consultancy perspectives.

What has impressed me recently is how approaches and methods previously identified with managers and management are now being eagerly taken-on and adopted for clinical leadership development. To take an example, Action Learning has part of its roots within healthcare, as Revans' pioneering work at Manchester Royal Infirmary reminds us (Revans, 1964), and has been employed in management development within the NHS for some years. It is also well-used in current managerial leadership development, as part of NHS Leadership Centre and NatPaCT programmes. More recently, however, Action Learning has been taken up as a means of jointly developing GPs and hospital consultants (see Jones & Wilson's chapter in this book); of providing continuing support to nurses and allied health professionals who have attended the LEO programme (see Dack's chapter); features prominently in the RCN Clinical Leadership programme (Cunningham and Mackenzie's chapter) and is being adopted by service improvement facilitators, risk management facilitators, collaborative project managers, etc – all of whom have emerged from a clinical professional background. That is not to say that Action Learning offers a leadership development panacea – Andrew Scowcroft's chapter points out the potential uses and abuses of the approach.

The time seems ripe, therefore, for a bringing-together of emerging practice in clinical leadership development within the NHS. The examples contained within this book are largely drawn from the NHS in England and Wales, not for any ethnocentric reasons (indeed, I am a Scot!), but because of the recent flowering of a wide diversity of development activity in and with the clinical professions there. I am sure that Scotland, and Northern Ireland also have tales to tell, but the contents inevitably reflect my own networks, connections and friendships. What central themes emerge from these accounts of clinical leadership development? There are some which seem fairly obvious and others which are perhaps less obvious but of greater import.

In the first category is the fact that increasingly clinical professionals see themselves as *leaders, rather than managers* – and actually prefer this distinction. It emerges most clearly in Thomas's chapter but runs as a current through many of the others. There is also the fact that although the stimulus for clinical leadership development can often be external (the NHS modernisation agenda (Inglis and Bevington); a Trust merger (Freer) or external accreditation requirements (Houghton)), the focus of much of the effort described here is what Julia Pokora and her colleagues call *"inside-out"* rather than "outside-in" development. It is not about the universal application of generic leadership competences, but rather is *individualised and holistic*, embracing personal and career development and employing a *multiplicity of development methods*, some of them based on development programmes, but others (Action Learning, coaching, shadowing, mentoring, succession planning, the use of the Soft Systems Methodology to elicit "Rich Pictures") much more work-based. This is essentially a clinical practitioner and manager viewpoint, as opposed to a Human Resources one (Gosling *et al.*, 2003).

Given the *representative* nature of much clinical leadership (see Chapter 1) it seems clear that NHS managers have generally avoided involvement in clinical leadership development – perhaps unsurprisingly, given the clinical professions preference for leadership rather than management, and it is obviously something that needs to be handled carefully and sensitively. As Peskett and King point out, however, this hands-off approach may be one of the causes of the polarised attitudes of "doctors in difficulty". A recent examination of clinical leadership in the Irish healthcare system (RCSI/IPA, 2003) also identified the absence of pre-existing effective working relationships with senior management as a major problem and identified a necessary foundation as "a supportive working relationship ... where mutual respect and trust are apparent". Jones and Wilson's chapter reveals what such creative engagement by chief executives can achieve. Another fascinating insight is the obvious enthusiasm and energy with which the case for *transformational leadership* is presented in the nursing, allied health professions and clinical scientists field (Cunningham & Mackenzie, Smith & Woodard) and the slightly cooler and more neutral observations of those who have conducted evaluation studies of such programmes (Griffiths *et al.*). Weaving together the multifarious clinical leadership programmes, projects and initiatives into something which makes sense locally and which has an *added-value or multiplier effect* is not easy, as Jan Freer' contribution illustrates.

The clinical leadership approaches described here are also powerfully *evidence-based,* employing a variety of diagnostics, such as the Kouzes and Posner Leadership Practices Inventory (Cunningham & Mackenzie); the Leadership Effectiveness Analysis™ (Dack, Houghton, Edmonstone) and Personal Directions™ (Edmonstone) all of which feature 360° feedback. For participants in such leadership development programmes this implies an openness to such feedback and an acceptance of the validity of the perceptions of significant others – their boss, staff and peers. Finally, it seems obvious that investment in clinical leadership development has proved quite liberating for many clinical professionals and has opened-up career opportunities which had not previously been dreamed off. A corollary of this, however, is that while such investment is welcomed, there is also a continuing concern (especially among the proponents of transformational leadership approaches) that empowerment of clinical leaders is not necessarily understood or accepted by some managerial leaders, who may find such challenges to their more traditional and transactional management practice to be potentially threatening.

At a more reflective level it is clear that our understanding of clinical leadership development is *incomplete* – this is a developing field with a number of exciting experiments taking place and with no single unified theory and practice in place. It is based upon a high degree of *uncertainty*, rather than total expertise. All the people who have contributed to this book would see themselves as continuously learning about developing clinical leaders. It is a *process* – "a journey rather than a destination" and involves:

- Seeking to understand and respond creatively to clinical professionals who take on leadership responsibilities.
- Learning by experiment and working to an extent by trial and error – but systematically reflecting on the experience and drawing-out useful theory which illustrates and explains action.
- Turning instincts and hunches into insight by thinking about what one is doing as one works and having an internal and external dialogue about such development work.

In this respect Andrew Scowcroft's chapter, which offers a series of reflections on the uses (and abuses) of Action Learning in leadership development offers a model for reflective practice for people in the clinical leadership development field. For clinical leadership development , like the work of clinical professionals ,is something which starts from *practice*. The hope is that this book will assist that process of discovery, encourage the dialogue and draw-out theory which is useful to others.

References

Attwood, M., Pedler, M., Pritchard, S. & Wilkinson, D. (2003) *Leading Change: A Guide to Whole System Working,* Bristol, The Policy Press.

Darwin, J., Johnson, P. & McAuley, J. (2002) *Developing Strategies for Change,* Harlow, Pearson Education.

Edmonstone, J. (1986) "If you're not the woodcutter, what are you doing with that axe?", *Health Services Manpower Review,* Vol. 12, No. 3, pp 8–12.

Fish, D. & Coles, C. (1998) *Developing Professional Judgement in Health Care: Learning Through the Critical Appreciation of Practice,* Oxford, Butterworth-Heinemann.

Gosling, S., Offley, N., Bristow, M. & Bailey, C. (2003) "Pushing rank", *Health Service Journal,* Supplement on Leadership (30th October).

Page, S. (1998) "Narrowing the gap between practice development and service management", in Page, S., Allsopp, D. & Casley, S. (eds), *The Practice Development Unit: An Experiment in Multidisciplinary Innovation,* London, Whurr.

Revans, R. (1964) *Standards for Morale in Hospitals,* London, Oxford University Press.

Royal College of Surgeons In Ireland/Institute of Public Administration (2003) *Clinicians in Management: A Review of Clinical Leadership,* Dublin, Office for Health Management.

CHAPTER ONE

What is clinical leadership development?

John Edmonstone

When Herbert Morrison was asked for a definition of socialism during the Attlee administration of 1945–51 he famously defined it as "What the Labour Government does". Adopting the same logic would lead to a conclusion that clinical leadership is simply what clinical professionals do when they lead! Yet such a simplistic statement hides as much as it reveals. The purpose of this chapter is therefore to describe the background or context within which leadership development in healthcare in the UK has developed; to compare and contrast clinical and managerial leadership; to review three main models of leadership (and some major questions which flow from them); to consider the range of development methods applicable to the development of clinical leaders, and finally to raise a number of major discussion points for the future of clinical leadership development.

Introduction

Historically, from the 1960s the NHS has spent millions of pounds on the training and development of *managers*, although the precise amount is unknown (Goodwin, 2000). Evaluation of such programmes has been largely non-robust and, at best, anecdotal. These programmes have focused primarily on individual managers (plus a small number of clinicians) from a range of different work settings and roles learning about management ideas and skills. Such programmes have sometimes been delivered by external providers (from within the Higher and Further Education systems) and sometimes on an in-house basis, and typically have offered little which was specific to the more local challenges facing individuals, groups or organisations. The creation of the NHS Leadership Centre in England has now led to an explosion in the number of *leadership* programmes targeted at specific groups of managers and clinicians and this is closely paralleled in Wales with the work of the Centre for Health Leadership. This development takes place against a backdrop of recurrent media attacks on NHS managers as "fat cats" and an increasingly sterile mantra of "White coats and stethoscopes: Good; Grey suits: Bad". Yet only some 3% of all NHS staff are managers and the proportion of total NHS expenditure consumed by management costs is only some 4%, compared with some 17% in the United States. Moreover, over 25% of NHS chief executives have moved to those positions from a clinical background (Carvel, 2003).

However, there may well be cause for concern as to whether this major investment in leadership development will pay real dividends and whether it is targeted appropriately. A major review of the business and health care literature (Vance & Larson, 2002) concluded that the search for a single definition of leadership seemed fruitless (and perhaps irrelevant), because an appropriate choice of definition depended upon the theoretical, methodological and substantive aspects of leadership being considered.

Most of the health care and business leadership literature which was reviewed consisted of anecdotal or theoretical discussions. Only 4.4% of 6,628 articles reviewed were data-based. The largest proportion of research (41.4%) was purely descriptive of demographic characteristics or the personality traits of leaders. Only 15.2% included any correlation of qualities or styles of leadership with measurable outcomes for service users or positive changes in organisations. They concluded that:

> "A great need exists for research focused on how leadership makes a difference in outcomes, such as quality patient care and improvements in organisational quality and productivity."

Knights or knaves?

This need to illustrate how investment in leadership development pays tangible dividends takes place against the growing emergence of two quite different models of health care (Davies & Harrison, 2002). On the one hand, there is the growing strength of what has been called the *"scientific-bureaucratic"* model which emphasises robust and objective evidence, formalised into prescriptions for clinical and managerial practice and advancing models for service delivery which serve to reduce individual discretion regarding patterns of clinical practice. This relates to what has been termed the "audit society" (Mearns *et al.*, 2003) with its

> "plethora of guidance, league tables, star-ratings, regulatory bodies and inspectorates, targets, national service frameworks, performance indicators, minimum standards, incentives and sanctions and regulations – all to cajole, coax, threaten, encourage, exhort and order public bodies to do the Government's bidding"
>
> Philpot, 2003

On the other hand, there is what is termed the *"reflective practice"* model in which the language and ideology of patient care is conceived on an individualised basis and clinical professionals tend (or seek) to work largely independently of the structural arrangements of their host organisation. This is paralleled by a growing polarisation between two views of professional practice, as noticed by Fish & Coles and shown in Table 1.1.

The Professional-Artistry approach tends to see the issue of fostering innovation in health care as complex, while the Technical-Rational approach sees it as merely complicated (Plsek, 2003), as shown in Table 1.2.

A range of developments over the last twenty years has served to strengthen the scientific-bureaucratic and technical-rational world-view at the expense of the reflective-practice and professional-artistry one. These include principally the 1990s attempt to create an internal market within the NHS and the associated "neo-unitary" philosophy, with:

- *A single source and locus of control* – general management
- *A single loyalty focus* – the employing organisation, not the profession
- *Common objectives* – through such means as mission statements, business plans, performance appraisal. (Edmonstone, 2003)

This is in direct contrast to earlier, more pluralistic, approaches – such as the notion that within human service organisations there were a number of distinct and self-sustaining "domains" which were simply loosely-coupled together (Edmonstone, 1982). These views are, in part, a continuing reflection of a debate which characterises public service

Table 1.1: Two views of professional practice (Fish & Coles, 1998)

Technical-rational view	Professional-artistry view
Follows rules, laws, routines and prescriptions	Starts where rules fade. Sees patterns and frameworks
Uses diagnosis and analysis	Uses interpretation and appreciation
Wants efficient systems	Wants creativity and room to be wrong
Sees knowledge as graspable and permanent	Sees knowledge as temporary, dynamic and problematic
Theory is applied to practice	Theory emerges from practice
Visible performance is central	There is more to it than surface features
Setting-out and testing for basic competency is vital	There is more to it than the sum of the parts
Technical expertise is all	Professional judgement counts
Sees professional activities as masterable	Sees mystery at the heart of professional activities
Emphasises the known	Embraces uncertainty
Standards must be fixed. They are measurable and must be controlled	That which is most easily fixed and measurable is also often trivial – professionals should be trusted
Emphasises assessment, performance appraisal, inspection and accreditation	Emphasises investigation, reflection and deliberation
Change must be managed from outside	Professionals can develop from inside
Quality is really about the quantity of that which is easily measurable	Quality comes from deepening insight into one's values, priorities and actions
Technical accountability	Professional answerability
Professionals should be trained for instrumental purposes	The development of professionals is intrinsically worthwhile

workers (and particularly professionals) as either self-interested egoists (who need to be carefully watched, regulated and controlled) – as "knaves"; or noble altruists, defending the public service ethos – as "knights" (Le Grand, 2003).

More recently the Bristol heart babies and Harold Shipman cases (and the ensuing strengthening of professional regulatory arrangements, the

Table 1.2: Contrasting approaches to innovation (Plsek, 2003)

Approach innovation as	Complicated	Complex
Underlying metaphor	Organisation as a machine – plan and control	Organisation as a complex adaptive system – learn and adapt as you go
Generation of ideas	Done by creative specialists and experts	Ideas can emerge from anyone, in any part of the system, at any time.
Implementation of ideas	Should be thoroughly planned out and be primarily a replication of structures and processes that have worked elsewhere	Can be informed by what has worked elsewhere, but needs to take into account local structures, processes and patterns
Widespread adoption across organisations	Primarily an issue of evidence, dissemination and motivation	Primarily an issue of sharing knowledge through social relationships and adapting ideas to fit local conditions
Receptive context for change	Health care organisations are largely similar and there are a small number of key issues that we must address to ensure success	Health care organisations are similar in some ways, but also have important unique characteristics that must be taken into account at times of change

advent of hospital consultant and GP appraisal, re-validation require-ments, etc) and the work of the Commission for Health Improvement as an inspectorial/advisory body have all served to strengthen the technical-rational and scientific-bureaucratic standpoint. While most clinical pro-fessionals can probably see the (political) rationale for the tightening and focusing of systems of appraisal, assessment, re-validation and "licensing", those same professionals would most probably also align their own per-sonal values closer to those of the reflective-practice and professional-artistry view. Yet, as has been pointed-out (Attwood *et al.*, 2003) most UK public service organisations do have more pluralistic cultures than many private sector enterprises, and so a key leadership challenge is to develop processes where people can learn to listen to and respect each other's perspectives across the divides of history, tradition, culture, edu-cation, previous experience, etc. Vibrant organisations tend to draw their strength from the different perspectives and beliefs held by professionals and managers and between people working at the "front-line" and those in central or headquarters positions. Diversity is valuable because innovation and learning are the product of such differences – no-one learns anything without being open to contrasting points of view (Heifitz & Laurie, 1997).

Clinical and managerial leadership

So what are the differences and similarities between clinical and managerial leadership? Historically, the focus of the former has typically been the *patient, client group or service*, while the focus of the latter has typically been more corporate, with the needs of the *organisation*. Yet this only takes us so far. Some years ago it was noted that, within managerial leadership systems, such leaders are appointed and operate within given policies and procedures in order to achieve targets. They are engaged in hierarchical manager-subordinate relationships with their "followers" who are managerially accountable to them (Jacques, 1976). Yet even here, a necessary precondition of effective leadership seems to be the degree of trust that is placed in the leader both by superiors and subordinates (Heifitz, 1994).

Such managerial leadership can be contrasted with so-called "elective" or representative leadership which starts from an essentially non-hierarchical premise – all members of a professional group are theoretically equal – and equally valuable. Debate, persuasion and negotiation are crucial if a consensus or majority view is to be reached within the professional group. Leadership in this setting is therefore about facilitating such debate, discussion and resultant action. Leaders require the social sensitivity to be able to "read" the emerging views of those whom they represent, and this is an "unconscious, accumulating judgement". Such leaders are either formally elected by their peers or informally "emerge" – but they remain *accountable to those who elected them*. Such elective leadership can be a fragile commodity (Plsek, 2003) and the incorporation of clinical leaders within an essentially managerial (hierarchical) framework runs the risk of diminishing the credibility of clinical leaders vis-à-vis their peers over time. Likewise, recent observations of such "non-corporate" forms of leadership (Wedderburn Tate, 1999) suggest that it is marked by the following characteristics:

- No formal leaders (leaders emerge out of events)
- A lack of formality between leaders and followers
- Leaders depend upon personal power (influence) rather than position or resource power
- The leadership role changes hands on several occasions
- There is scope for confusion, factionalism and divided loyalties
- Leaders tend to be more charismatic
- There are few structures or procedures.

Clinical leadership can best be described as *leadership by clinicians of clinicians*. *Clinician* in this context means all health professionals, including doctors, nurses, midwives and allied health professions. *Clinical leaders* are all those who still retain a clinical role, but at the same time take a significant part in direction-setting, resource management, motivation of colleagues, etc. It does not include clinicians who have become full-time managers (Wright *et al.*, 2001). Leadership is therefore not something separate from clinical practice, but "a continuous and everyday activity that is an explicit part of all senior clinical roles" (Detmer & Ford, 2001). A recent review of clinical leadership within the healthcare system of Ireland (RCSI/IPA, 2003) suggested that a "common thread" for all clinical leaders embodied:

- The use of persuasion rather than hierarchical power to change peoples' attitudes and behaviour.
- The use of evidence to make the case for change to managers and professional colleagues.
- The provision of "case studies" or exemplars of successful change to get colleagues on board.
- The advance preparation of major change by consultation and clarification, anticipating problems and providing options.

The study concluded that the credibility and acceptability of clinical leaders rested upon their ability to act as advocates for patient care and clinical service developments, rather than simply being seen as the "clinical arm of executive management".

On this basis the chairs of Professional Executive Committees (PECs) of Primary Care Trusts (PCTs), the chairs of Local Medical Committees

(LMCs) of GPs, the chairs of councils of those Trusts operating a system of Shared Governance and the co-ordinators of integrated self-managing community nursing teams would all be such elective leaders. Clinical Directors in Acute hospital settings are typically appointed by their chief executive and/or medical director, but would need to have the support of the clinicians within the specialty (or group of specialties) which they represent – so are perhaps a "hybrid" form.

Attempts at innovation based solely within the formal managerial system of health care, defined by hierarchical boss-subordinate relationships can be aided or thwarted by interactions within the more informal "shadow systems" of clinical leadership (Plsek, 2003). Any chief executive ignoring or wishing-away this reality is quite clearly short-sighted!

Approaches to leadership

A recent review (Walker, 2002) identified three major approaches to leadership – trait theories, contingency and style theories and transformational leadership.

1. *Trait theories* reflect the notion that leaders behave in particular ways because of particular *personal characteristics* or *psychological dispositions*. They assume that good leaders can be defined or described by the traits which they have in common and see leadership as a definable commodity or set of skills with a high degree of generality across professions, organisations, sectors of the economy or society, and even across countries (Heifitz, 1994). It has been claimed that the trait-based approach results from a form of "naïve reductionism" where the means to understanding things is to reduce them to their component parts, rather than seeing them holistically and in an emergent fashion (Wilson & Chesterman, 2003). Such a viewpoint also tends to deny a place for values. The basic idea behind this essentially "psychologistic" approach (that leadership traits exist *within* individuals) remains both influential and popular – most methods for selecting people for leadership positions (such as the NHS graduate-entry Management Training Scheme) rely heavily on trait leadership assumptions and most competency-based approaches to leadership also follow this assumption. Unfortunately, the trait-based approach also serves to

reproduce the "great man" theory of history, with a heavily-gendered emphasis. The dangers of existing managerial leadership in the NHS simply "cloning" itself has been noted (Alimo-Metcalfe, 1999) and more recently the dangers of "homophily" have been recognised (Faugier & Woolnough, 2001). This is defined as:

> "The tendency to work or interact with people who are similar demographically or attitudinally."

and suggests that when the majority of leaders in any organisation is made up of one demographic group (such as white men of a certain age) and when decisions about promotion are based (even in part) on their preference for working with people who are demographically similar – we can say that a significant bias has entered the advancement process.

2. *Contingency and style theories* suggest that what matters is matching *leadership behaviour* to *situational demands*. Effectiveness is not seen to be directly associated with a particular leadership style and will produce different outputs according to different circumstances. The shift is from traits to behaviour – so encouraging the notion that leadership can be developed rather than simply identified and selected. The model of situational leadership (Blanchard, Hershey & Johnson, 1996) which forms a significant element of the Leading an Empowered Organisation (LEO) programme is derived from this approach.

3. **Transformational leadership** is founded on the notion that innovative, inspirational and proactive leaders with the ability to motivate others to pursue high standards and long-term goals are needed to achieve the kinds of changes envisaged in the NHS Plan – "to strive beyond the ordinary to achieve the exceptional". It is claimed that transformational leaders recognise that in order to deliver high quality patient care, an empowering culture needs to be created where communication, strong values (including a powerful belief in human potential), a tolerance of mistakes and mutual respect are paramount (Clegg, 2000). This is contrasted with transactional management, with an emphasis on planning, budgeting, organising and controlling in order to achieve goals. The LEO programme mentioned above reflects transformational

leadership values, and the use of value-based diagnostics derived from transformational leadership models (Kouzes & Posner, 1995) is also central to the RCN Clinical Leadership Development Programme (Cunningham & Kitson, 1997, 2000a, 2000b).

Emerging questions

A number of pertinent question about clinical leadership in the NHS emerge from a consideration of these approaches. It has been suggested, for example (Goodwin, 2000), that it is increasingly inappropriate to concentrate on an *individual's* ability to lead and that there is, instead, a need to develop a "local leadership mindset". In a similar vein, in research conducted by the NHS Leadership Centre which sought to identify the contribution that chief executives made to their organisation's "star-rating" (Dawes, 2002) it was suggested that chief executives were not actually significant in changing the performance of their organisation and posited that they had very little to do with how their organisation as a whole functioned. Such a perspective certainly challenges taken-for-granted assumptions about the relationship between chief executives and leadership within organisations and again shifts the focus from leadership as a characteristic of individuals to that of an *organisational capacity*. It raises the prospect that leadership is not something that rests in a few talented individuals, but is an aspect of the whole organisation – and thus reflects how teams support each other, learn from mistakes and instigate service change. Leadership is thus seen as being something "for the many, not the few." Such a viewpoint is also supported by Senge (1997) who claims that in the future it will be necessary to surrender the myth of leaders as isolated heroes and to replace it with leadership distributed among diverse individuals and teams sharing responsibility for creating an organisation's future.

This idea of the importance of a leadership mind-set or "gestalt" embodies the assumptions of shared (or distributed) leadership (Edmonstone *et al.*, 2003) that:

• *Effective leadership can and should be present at all levels in an organisation.* It is not confined to the people at the "top", but permeates all areas.

- *There is no single "one right way" to lead.* The diversity and complexity of people, organisations, challenges and opportunities are too great to allow for one approach that works in all situations.
- *Effective leadership is based on behaviour* – the ability to "make and mend" relationships in order to facilitate performance, co-operation, production and mutual job satisfaction.
- *Effective leadership is situational.* There are many roads to leadership effectiveness and the path taken will depend on the demands of the specific situations individuals and groups find themselves in.

Shared leadership finds organisational expression in such phenomena as multidisciplinary team-working (Borrill *et al.*, 2001) and in structural arrangements designed to support Shared Governance (Edmonstone, 2003). Interestingly enough, the extent of investment in these areas has been minimal in comparison with the more individual-based leadership development programmes instigated at national and local levels.

Three major barriers to leadership development in the NHS have been identified (Alimo-Metcalfe & Alban-Metcalfe, 2003). They are:

- That top managers believe that their status in the organisation is evidence enough that they "have what it takes" to be regarded as a leader and so regard their ongoing development as unnecessary – although the managers "below" them certainly need it.
- That managers returning from leadership development experiences become more aware of the poor quality of the leadership role-modelled by more senior managers – and their frustration levels increase.
- That the suggestions made by such returnees are either rejected or ignored.

These processes serve to provoke disenchantment, greater cynicism and lower morale. Although Alimo-Metcalfe and Alban-Metcalfe are describing managerial leaders, where investment is made in clinical leadership development, these dangers also exist – but this time with larger numbers of front-line staff. The evaluation study of the LEO programme (Woolnough & Faugier, 2002) commented:

"If senior staff fail to offer their support, the result will be a cadre of nurse leaders disempowered and disillusioned by their capacity to make changes."

and this message was further amplified by those close to the design and development of the LEO programme itself (Garland *et al.*, 2002):

"Clinical leaders returning with new skills and ideas have a right to expect an organisation that is willing to change to accommodate those ideas. That is the real nature of the contract entered into by participation in the national clinical leadership programme. Continuing to condone organisational practices that punish, control access to information, align responsibility with title rather than ability and limit decision-making to a select few will risk alienating one of the most valuable assets of the NHS – its clinical leaders."

A recent long-term research study on innovation conducted by Roffey Park Institute (Shelton & Syrett, 2003) suggested that in healthcare the biggest fallacy was that *managers* alone felt obligated to originate creative thinking that leads to innovation, rather than to identify, champion and support it. They suggest that managers are not "mandated" to undertake this supportive role and that, indeed, it is discretionary for them (either because they feel they are paid to "know it all" or because they are preoccupied with short-term targets and more immediate corporate priorities) – and thus shy-away from promoting new thinking.

Leadership development methods

The "programmatic" nature of leadership development in the NHS (see below) was identified and critiqued by evaluation studies of programmes for executive directors run in two former NHS regions in the late 1990s (Edmonstone & Western, 2002). As a result, work-based approaches (Raelin, 2000) have become more popular. These involve learning from another person, learning from tasks and learning with others and are shown in Table 1.3 (based on Woodall & Winstanley, 1999):

There is a very real danger of "fashion swings" in which leadership development moves between programmatic and course-based approaches on the one hand and work-based alternatives on the other (and then back again!), while in all likelihood a judicious mix of such methods is probably the most effective way forward.

Table 1.3: Work-based development methods

Methods	Learning progress
Learning from another person	
Coaching	Feedback, reflection & challenge
Mentoring	Support, advice, feedback, opportunity and challenge
Role models	Observation, reflection and imitation
Learning from tasks	
Special projects	Problem-solving, taking responsibility, taking risks and making decisions
Job rotation	Exposure to other cultures and viewpoints
Shadowing	Observation of tasks, new techniques and skills
Secondment	Exposure to other cultures and viewpoints
Acting-up	Trial of new tasks and skills, challenges
Learning with others	
Task forces and working parties	Strategic understanding, building awareness and confidence
Action learning	Problem-solving, interaction, influencing
Networking	Interaction and building awareness

The future of clinical leadership development

Clinical leadership development is such a recent phenomenon that it seems strange to be raising questions about the future. Yet the experience so far (much of which is captured in this book) suggests that there are at least three major issues to be resolved.

The first relates to the distinction made between *transactional and transformational leadership.* The latter is undoubtedly much more attractive and "sexy" than the former although everyone recognises that both are needed in practice. There is undoubtedly a degree of scepticism among both clinicians and managers as to whether, given the highly-politicised nature of the NHS, the rhetoric about "earned autonomy", decentralisation and empowerment is actually real. The legacy of centralised command-and-control has proved stubbornly resistant to change because the strong political imperatives for retaining central direction of the NHS remain (Robinson, 2002).

However, even if this does prove to be the direction of travel, it raises questions about where and in what numbers transactional and transformational leaders are needed. Some years ago Charles Handy developed a model of organisations which suggested that while some areas of the enterprise were concerned with innovation before anything else (and where in today's terms transformational leadership would be appropriate), other parts of an organisation were concerned with "steady-state" activities, where transactional leadership would seem to provide a better "fit" (Handy, 1976). Greater attention may be needed to the work-settings and the drivers within them which lead to requirements for particular types of leadership.

The 1990s evaluation studies of leadership development programmes (Edmonstone & Western, 2002) highlighted a form of "conceptual fuzziness" with regard to the transactional/transformational issue (amongst others) and this also translates into the design and content of national leadership programmes. For example, the LEO and RCN Clinical Leadership programmes are quite clearly value-based and transformational in nature – and explicitly so. The RCN programme makes use of the Leadership Practices Inventory (LPI), a diagnostic instrument derived from the "five fundamental practices of exemplary leadership" (Kouzes & Posner, 1995). Yet the national Medical Leadership programmes take a much lower-key view of such matters and feature another diagnostic tool (the Myers-Briggs Type Instrument or MBTI) as a key stimulus to self-insight among programme participants. Quite what the rationale is for these important differences is not particularly clear. What is clear is that these different "sub-texts" do not make the integration of such divergent streams of national investment at a local level any easier.

This leads to the second issue – that of the domination of a *programmatic rather than a contextual approach*. Programmatic approaches are based on distinct "episodes" with a clear beginning, middle and end, and "bracketed-off" from ongoing organisational life (Edmonstone, 1995), and in this sense the national leadership development effort can largely be said to be programmatic. There were over 20 national programmes sponsored by the NHS Leadership Centre identifiable in early 2003. By contrast, the contextual approach (Pettigrew *et al.*, 1992) suggests that development is a dynamic, non-linear and local process and places emphasis on both external (political and economic) and internal (history, culture, social networks) factors.

It has been noted (Wilkinson & Appelbee, 1999) that the public services are dominated by the programmatic approach, which assumes that organisations are like machines and can be "fixed" by top-down imposed change. The instigators of programmatic change efforts are typically top management and human resource staff – rarely local clinical professionals or managers. Programmatic initiatives are experienced as:

> "led by different individuals, detached from each other and divorced from any connecting bigger picture"
>
> Wilkinson & Appelbee, 1999

There is thus a major problem for organisations in capitalising on and integrating the efforts of national programmes in a local context in order to add value. A contextualist approach would not discount the value of leadership development programmes, but would place the emphasis firmly on how well (with what results) such leadership was exercised within the local organisational or network context. This emphasis on context also reflects the view that leadership resides not *in* individuals, but in the human relationships *between* individuals (and their organisations) — and simply cannot be reduced easily to a set of traits or behaviours (Heifitz, 1994). A recent review of programmatic approaches to leadership development in Further Education (Wilson & Chesterman, 2003) also argued for a shift of emphasis away from individual skills and towards collective leadership processes or "institutional development". To be fair to the NHS Leadership Centre, it would appear that they are now determined to re-align leadership development much more along contextual than programmatic lines, although their "inheritance" most likely makes this an incremental rather than a dramatic change.

A third issue relates to whether leadership development activity is actually *preparing people for the future*, rather than the present or past. One recent and major feature of health care has been the development of managed clinical networks in cancer, coronary heart disease and other services. In such networks the skills required seem to be largely those of a diplomat –the ability to influence and negotiate (Ferlie & Pettigrew, 1996). The skills needed to work in such settings are said to include:

- *Trading* across professional, organisational, social and political boundaries.

- *Broking* – the ability to see the big picture, make connections, be credible to different groups and to broker partnerships.
- *Persuading* – strong interpersonal, communication and listening skills; the ability to act as an interpreter and a sense-maker; the ability to mediate, arbitrate and manage conflict.
- *Facilitating* – the ability to animate relationships between network members, together with teaching, dissemination, mentoring and knowledge-transfer skills.
- *Learning* – a high tolerance of ambiguity and uncertainty; the ability to reflect on and conceptualise experience and the ability to learn quickly, adapting to changing situations. (Pedler, 2001)

It would be heartening to know that leadership development programmes were preparing people for such a future setting. Additionally, many services (particularly mental health, learning disabilities, older people and children) now have to be delivered in a whole-system and partnership fashion and it is noteworthy that health leadership development in Scotland tends to take place in a public sector-wide framework, under the aegis of the Scottish Leadership Foundation. Recent developments in England by the Integrated Care Network suggest that multi-agency programmes are increasingly seen as the way forward.

The early years of the 21st century have seen a flowering of clinical leadership development in health care. The number of initiatives, programmes, etc can seem overwhelming and is redolent of Mao Ze Duong's enjoinder to:

> "Let a thousand flowers blossom. Let a thousand schools of thought contend."

Greater sense-making and focus would seem to be needed to take clinical leadership development into an uncertain future.

References.

Alimo-Metcalfe, B. (1999) "Leadership in the NHS: what are the competencies and qualities needed and how can they be developed?", in Mark, A. & Dopson, S. (eds.), *Organisational Behaviour in Health Care: The Research Agenda*, London, Macmillan.

Alimo-Metcalfe, B. & Alban-Metcalfe, J. (2003) "Stamp of greatness", *Health Service Journal* (26 June), pp 28–32.

Attwood, M., Pedler, M., Pritchard, S. & Wilkinson, D. (2003) *Leading Change: A Guide to Whole Systems Working,* Bristol, The Policy Press.

Blanchard, K., Hershey, P. & Johnson D. (1996) *Management of Organisational Behaviour,* 7th edition, New Jersey, Prentice-Hall.

Borrill, C., Carletta, J., Carter, A., Dawson, J., Garrod, S., Rees, A., Richards, A., Shapiro, D. & West, M. (2001) *The Effectiveness of Health Care Teams in the NHS,* Aston University/University of Glasgow/University of Edinburgh/ University of Leeds.

Carvel, J. (2003) "Team talk", *Guardian,* 25th June.

Clegg, A (2000) "Leadership: improving the quality of patient care", *Nursing Standard,* Vol. 14, No. 30, pp 43–45.

Cunningham, G. & Kitson, A. (2000a) "An evaluation of the RCN Clinical Leadership Development Programme: Part 1", *Nursing Standard,* Vol. 15, No. 2, pp 34–37.

Cunningham, G. & Kitson, A. (2000b) "An evaluation of the RCN Clinical Leadership Development Programme: Part 2", *Nursing Standard,* Vol. 15, No. 3, pp 34–40.

Cunningham, G. & Kitson, A. (1997) *Ward Leadership Project: A Journey to Patient-Centred Leadership,* Executive Summary, London, Royal College of Nursing.

Davies, H. & Harrison, S.(2002) "Trends in doctor–manager relationships", *bmj.com.*

Dawes, D. (2002) "Stars of wonder", *Health Service Journal* (12 September), pp 26–27.

Detmer, D. & Ford, J. (2001) "Educating leaders for healthcare", *Clinician in Management,* No. 10, pp 3–5.

Edmonstone, J. (2003) *Shared Governance: Making it Happen*, Chichester, Kingsham Press.

Edmonstone, J. (1995) "Managing change: an emerging new consensus", *Health Manpower Management,* Vol. 21, No. 1, pp 16–19.

Edmonstone, J. (1982) "Human service organisations: implications for management and organisation development", *Management Education & Development,* Vol. 13, Part 3, pp 163–173.

Edmonstone, J. & Western, J. (2002) "Leadership development in health care: what do we know?", *Journal of Management in Medicine,* Vol. 16, No. 1, pp 34–47.

Edmonstone, J., Hamer, S. & Smith, S. (2003) "Integrated community nursing teams: an evaluation study", *Community Practitioner,* Vol. 76, No. 10, pp 386–389.

Faugier, J. & Woolnough, H. (2001) "Breaking the male mould: a new approach to leadership", *Mental Health Practice,* Vol. 4, No. 9 (June).

Ferlie, E. & Pettigrew, A. (1996) "Managing through networks: some issues and implications for the NHS", *British Journal of Management,* No. 7, pp 581–589.

Fish, D. & Coles, C. (1998) *Developing Professional Judgement in Health Care: Learning Through the Critical Appreciation of Practice,* Oxford, Butterworth-Heinemann.

Garland, G., Smith, S. & Faugier, J. (2002) "Supporting clinical leaders in achieving organisational change", *Professional Nurse,* Vol. 17, No. 8, pp 490–492.

Goodwin, N. (2000) "The National Leadership Centre and the National Plan", *British Journal of Health Care Management,* Vol. 6, No. 9, pp 399–401.

Handy, C. (1976) *Understanding Organisations,* Harmondsworth, Penguin.

Heifitz, R. (!994) *Leadership Without Easy Answers,* Cambridge, MA, Belknap Press.

Heifitz, R. & Laurie, D. (1997) "The work of leadership", *Harvard Business Review,* Vol. 75, No. 1 (January/February), pp 124–134.

Jacques, E. (1976) *A General Theory of Bureaucracy,* London, Heinemann.

Kouzes, & Posner, B. (1995) *The Leadership Challenge: How to Keep Getting Extraordinary Things Done in Organisations,* San Francisco, Jossey-Bass.

Le Grand, J. (2003) *Motivation, Agency and Public Policy: of Knights and Knaves, Pawns and Queens,* London, Oxford University Press.

Mearns, R., Richards, S. & Smith, R. (2003) *Community Care: Policy and Practice,* 3rd Edition, Basingstoke, Palgrave-Macmillan.

Pedler, M. (2001) *Networked Organisations: an Overview,* Health Development Agency.

Pettigrew, A., Ferlie, E. & McKee, L. (1992) *Shaping Strategic Change: Managing Change in Large Organisations: the Case of the National Health Service,* London, Sage.

Philpot, T. (2003) "Planned on the run", *Health Service Journal,* Vol. 113, No. 5880, p. 21.

Plsek, P. (2003) *Complexity and the Adoption of Innovation in Health Care,* National Institute for Health Care Management Foundation/National Committee For Quality Health Care.

Royal College of Surgeons In Ireland/Institute of Public Administration (2003) *Clinicians in Management: A Review of Clinical Leadership,* Discussion Paper 4, Dublin, Office For Health Management.

Raelin, J. (2000) *Work-Based Learning: the New Frontier of Management Development,* New Jersey, Prentice-Hall.

Robinson, R. (2002) "Who's got the master card?", *Health Service Journal,* (26 September), pp 22–24.

Senge, P. (1997) "Communities of leaders and learners in looking ahead: implications of the present", *Harvard Business Review,* (September–October), pp 18–32.

Shelton, P. & Syrett, M. (2003) "Whose bright idea?", *Health Service Journal,* Vol. 113, No. 5883, pp 26–27.

Vance, C. & Larson, E. (2002) "Leadership research in business and health care", *Journal of Nursing Scholarship,* Vol. 34, No. 2, pp 165–171.

Walker, R. (2002) *Building Capacity For Developmental Evaluation,* Elliott-Walker Consultancy for West Yorkshire Workforce Development Confederation.

Wedderburn Tate, C. (1999) *Leadership in Nursing,* London, Churchill Livingstone.

Wilkinson, D. & Appelbee, E. (1999) *Implementing Holistic Government: Joined-up Action on the Ground,* Bristol, The Policy Press.

Wilson, P. & Chesterman, D. (2003) "Schools of leadership", *Organisations & People,* Vol. 10, No. 3 (August), pp 23–28.

Woodall, J. & Winstanley, D. (1999) *Management Development: Strategy and Practice,* Oxford, Blackwell.

Woolnough, H. & Faugier, J. (2002) "An evaluative study assessing the impact of leading an empowered organisation programme", *NT Research*, Vol. 7, No. 6, pp 412–427.

Wright, L., Malcolm, L., Barnett, P. & Hendry, C. (2001) *Clinical Leadership and Clinical Governance: A Review of Developments in New Zealand and Internationally,* Clinical Leaders Association of New Zealand for New Zealand Ministry of Health.

CHAPTER TWO

Medical leadership: doctors, the state and prospects for improvement

Calum Paton, David Whitney and Jenny Cowpe

Leadership – within, of and without medicine – is squarely on the agenda of the NHS. The Government's ambitious plans for service improvement within the NHS are driven by the need to satisfy more active citizens and demanding "consumers". Only then will a tax-funded NHS (the fairest and most cost-effective model) (DoH, 2000) be politically sustainable in the long term. Such improvement requires leadership for and by clinicians.

Accordingly, the changing relationship between doctors and the state is partly based on the fact that the earlier, informal "deal" between the two (see Part 1 below) must now take account of a more informed and (sometimes) sceptical public. Doctors are still trusted highly by comparison with other occupational groups. They are also still powerful, although losing autonomy of a certain sort at the edges. Yet the challenge now is to harness this professional power and authority to a collective agenda based on the highest clinical standards and the appropriate use of resources – standards and criteria developed to a large extent through the professional expertise of doctors.

Part 1 of this chapter explores the political economy underlying the changing relationship between doctors and the state. Part 2 outlines briefly how the recent history of "medical management" has brought us to the current situation. Part 3 then sets out the rationale for the Medical Leadership Programme which has been directed and co-ordinated from Keele University's Centre for Health Planning and Management and explores some issues arising for the future – which in some cases can be related to issues raised in Parts 1 and 2.

PART 1: DOCTORS AND THE STATE

Doctors, the state and political economy

The unwritten and informal "deal" between the state and doctors before 1991 meant that the doctors did not seriously question overall resources or their public-sector pay, and therefore did the rationing (Moran, 1999). However, they did it their way, in the context of professional and clinical autonomy and also with ill-defined private sector opportunities via an ill-defined public contract. The proposed new consultant contract in 2002 and the amended version agreed in October 2003, between Secretary of State for Health and the British Medical Association was geared to reversing the informal deal – doctors would get more money in return for (in some senses) less autonomy. The underlying sources of diminished autonomy are of course multiple, not least public expectations and go well beyond the immediate politics of the "consultant contract". Doctors will still regulate themselves, within developing national standards. Yet "inspection" will monitor such self-regulation. Doctors will still do (some of) the rationing, yet they will do so in the context of national and local targets and priorities, and so their freedom will be circumscribed. These issues are explored further below.

There may well now be convergence between the state's (and public) expectations and the central policy agenda. Research has suggested (Feachem *et al.*, 2002) that the "success" of Kaiser Permanente in California is related both to doctors' behaviour and (possibly) to medical leadership. More comprehensive and convenient primary care services for Kaiser patients go alongside more rapid access to more generously-provided specialist services and hospital admissions. In a nutshell, Kaiser employs more and better-paid specialists by comparison with the NHS as a "quid pro quo" for more effective management for in-patient time (with fewer days resulting) and the interfaces between primary, secondary and post-secondary care. Without more effective joint leadership by "managers" and doctors, it is difficult to see this happening. Although some of the research's methodology may be questioned, British Health Ministers were seriously interested in "trialling" the Kaiser approach in the UK, although this has not yet happened. Indeed the Primary Care Trust/hospital separation may thus be a step in the wrong direction.

Paradoxically, when money was tighter in the "old" NHS (between 1948 and the early 1990s), although fairly complete autonomy for the medical profession was the political price of under-funding, it was never-theless true that under-funding also meant that "autonomy" could be burdensome. In other words, even "doing the rationing our own way" could be irksome for the doctors. Governments needed doctors to have enough autonomy so that tough decisions were not unequivocally placed at Government's door, either by doctors or the public. Doctors might want autonomy in theory, yet get fed up with it in practice; whereas Governments will always rely on (partial) medical autonomy! There has always, therefore, been an unwelcome element to "autonomy" for the medical profession, under conditions of scarcity. The welcome element, conversely, has been freedom from centrally-set targets, in the past, so that limited funds will at least be applied by doctors' own decisions. Yet even this can be overestimated as a source of "past tranquility". The real-ity has always been that, with resources constrained, some specialties will win and others lose. Clinical autonomy presented a mixed picture for (different elements of) the medical profession.

The "new devolution" is about "empowering" doctors at the front line i.e. co-opting them! More money for the NHS may mean *less* of a politi-cal need for medical autonomy, but will allow actually *more* autonomy at the level of service and decision-making for individual patients, as long as that autonomy is in line with clinical governance. That way, doctors can still carry, or at least share, the burden of tough decisions. This is a very British "managed care", a kind of kinder, gentler Kaiser Permanente! For the future, however, it is a way forward, for it allows self-regulation by the profession as long as standards and outcomes are met. (Incidentally, one version of the "Foundation Trust" model seems to cut right across this – promoting as it does "consumer control" by the local community rather than the more sensible "producer control"). The key contrast with the past is that – following the developments outlined in Part 2 – priority-set-ting within Trusts, which should certainly involve medical leaders at its core, is on the basis of evidence-based "business plans" rather than the politics of the pig trough.

In the early NHS, the policy was universalism and comprehensiveness; and both limited technology and political economy allowed this part-laudable fact, part-fiction to apply. Medical possibilities were more limited; and in terms of political economy we were in the era of the industrial welfare state. As a result, the state did not have to invest selectively in niche industries and services to ensure international competitiveness (Jessop, 2002). The welfare state helped capitalism reproduce itself through social investment, to be distinguished from social expenses (O'Connor, 1973.) That was, however, chickenfeed compared to today's "competition state" which makes the state less autonomous, less a guarantor of universalism and yet more complex in its economic role (Paton, 2000).

What rationing was necessary was done informally, by doctors acting within the state's distribution of resources (both primary and specialised) ... for example, GPs would "turn away" the elderly for kidney transplants by custom and practice or would turn away those for whom hospital referral was a tall order due to local lack of provisions, unsuitability for travel, etc.

That is, implementing policy fitted-in with the unwritten grand design of policy – the noble lie, if you like.

Nowadays, the policy is both to invest in the economy in the context of global capitalism, *and* to ensure responses to consumerism and demands for higher quality, by no means just by the middle-classes, although more by them. This necessitates more money and more intensive use of resources, including human.

Implementation of such a strategy means that doctors and others must be "on board" (as managers would put it) regarding priorities and whom to prioritise ... otherwise firms will not get what they need from the NHS and/or the public won't. *And if this is so, then either firms will make greater use of private occupational healthcare and/or individuals will use the private sector more. Either way, the tax base of the NHS will be undermined, as firms and individuals are less willing to pay for a service that does not deliver what they want.*

And if doctors and others are "on board" with the NHS's mission to invest in the workforce, then economically less central strata in society may find that the NHS's relative exit from general care and rescue makes it less appealing to them.

Thus, to have the active support (as opposed to the sullen acquiescence) of the worse-off and less economically productive, the NHS must be fair and universal. To have the support of the middle-classes as consumers, it must be a modern service of three or preferably four-star quality and hotel status. To have the support of industry, it must provide a healthy workforce at economical cost.

Hence the ambitiousness of the NHS Plan!

The causes of doctors' disillusionment

Priorities for expenditure within the NHS are affected by the economic regime. A mass production and mass consumption society is consonant with mass welfare. In a society where greater economic and social differentiation has occurred, different strata among the "better-off" will have higher, and less homogeneous, expectations of health services, public or private. There will be pressure for the state's role to change from direct provision on an egalitarian, universalist basis to "investing in the profitable" i.e. to ensuring that potentially successful economic niches are supported. This is part of what some characterise as "post Fordism" (Clegg, 1990).

Today, the medical profession is confronting (partial and limited) de-professionalisation and proletarianisation. Regarding the latter, the doctor as individual entrepreneur/producer or craftsman is being superseded. Regarding the former, both the content of work and the organization of work is increasingly controlled (or at least influenced) by external actors such as the public and the state. This leaves clinically excellent doctors who are politically naïve or resentful of these changes belligerent or pessimistic, or both.

Next, like all worthy professions, there is conservatism within it – sometimes a force for good, sometimes not. This may be allied to what comes over sometimes as arrogance, born of both social and medical culture and the "exceptionalism" imparted through medical education and sense of mission.

Next, there are idealists who oppose "target-it is" and its effects, just as there were idealists who opposed the internal market in the 1990s – on moral and intellectual grounds which are not easily challenged!

Next, there are those who act from self-interest, specialty-interest and cadre-interest, (heavily but not exclusively economic interest). It is here that the first (rejected) version of the new consultant contract is interesting. While the contract had its rigidities (e.g. evening and Saturday morning work as part of the contract was a red rag to a bull out of proportion to its likely salience) the basic deal was that those who were substantially and largely committed to the NHS would benefit, whereas those who wanted to (continue to) indulge significantly in private work would see (over time) less (relative) remuneration and career progression in the public sector.

For those for whom private work was non-existent or marginal, this should or could have been seen as a means of increasing equity in reward (e.g. paediatricians as against orthopaedic surgeons!) But the minority who supported the original contract found that *their* economic self-interest was supplanted by a generalised negativity among different cadres and specialties. This spread, under the banner of disillusionment with the Government. Even those who might have benefited focused on the threats or rigidities in the contract.

More pragmatically, those consultants who were genuinely working hard hours – due to manpower shortages in many specialities, some acutely so; to Working Time Directives from Europe; and to post-Calman education which left both training-grade doctors and more junior consultants less "productive" at the coalface – saw little scope for "more contribution" to the NHS. Here, money was not (necessarily) the issue – although some such doctors might have received "more for the same" under the new contract.

The acceptance of the second version of the contract was based on a political compromise – but a creative one, auguring quite well for an improving relationship between doctors and the state (and hopefully one based upon a new consensus both as to priorities and to the need to avoid "control freakery" and micro-management by the state, although there is a long way to go).

The policy and leadership challenge

In opposition by the mid-1990s, Labour had a surprising honeymoon with the medical profession, and even or especially the BMA under the leadership of Dr Sandy Macara. Perhaps not so surprising – many doctors opposed the internal market, but for varying reasons. Some were bona fide believers in an altruistic public service; some objected to the bureaucracy without clear results, the "much ado about nothing" aspect of the internal market. Some were losers, pure and simple, in a more transparent business planning; others were losers because "priorities" crowded out their services. Some resented the increased, although circumscribed, power for managers; and some were Mr. Blair's "forces of conservatism", reactionaries who didn't mind attacks upon "professions" as long as it wasn't theirs!

Labour's honeymoon, in office, was soon over. Equally predictable, in one way – but it need not have led to such acrimonious divorce so soon. Labour's worthwhile ideological challenge was to stress outcomes and quality in a renewed NHS, but in the context of a dismantling of the "command-and-control" healthcare state i.e. the state it inherited from Mrs. Thatcher. Instead it has continued and deepened the "control state".

Part 2 below outlines how we got to the present situation.

PART 2: THE RECENT HISTORY OF MEDICAL LEADERSHIP

What were the origins and foundations of doctors becoming involved in clinical management? How has this role evolved and developed over the past two decades and what future direction will it take?

In 1974 'consensus management' was developed in the NHS. Its origins lay in work done by Professor Elliot Jacques and his team at Brunel University arising, in part, from their work with the Glacier Metal Company (Jaques, 1978). The Area and District Management Teams comprised doctors, administrators, nurses, treasurers and (perhaps) a representative of the local medical school. The Chair of the District Management Team was held on a rotating basis annually.

This was the first formal introduction of the word "management" to the NHS, but none of the senior participants in the District Management Team (DMT) had that word in their job title and the culture of consensus management sometimes meant that agreement was on the basis of "lowest common denominator" decisions. Consensus of opinion within the team could mean creative compromise or even genuine agreement based on altruism as well as sectional interest – but where agreement was impossible, the DMT would have to refer its agenda "upwards" to the Board (at Area level until 1982, then at District level).

Consensus management can be interpreted as a milestone along the evolutionary path towards general management within the NHS. Others however see it as an alternative model – and, internationally, its advantages as well as disadvantages have been perceived.

DMT meetings considered financial and patient activity at some level of detail but only at macro-level across the organisation. At the same time the Health Service was operating the "Cogwheel" machinery of medical administration whereby each specialty had its own Division comprising medical consultants within that specialty, electing their own Chair and being supported by a Cogwheel Medical Administrator. Their deliberations were recorded in a set of minutes that went to the DMT meetings either for information or to alert the DMT of an issue that they wish to have considered. The "Cogwheel" meetings were an early form of clinical directorates within the NHS, but with one fundamental difference – they had no resources to manage. The reason for this was that the DMT did not have the ability to separate-out its global budget into specific specialty budgets such as orthopaedics and radiology. The technique of specialty costing emerged during the early 1980's through the NHS Resource Management Initiative, which sought to apportion the budget for the whole organisation. This was the real driver and incentive for doctors to get involved in management – they had resources to manage and financial and patient activity information to support them in doing so.

These developments went hand-in-hand with the establishment of the Griffiths Inquiry (in 1982, reporting in October 1983) into the management of the NHS by the Conservative Government of the day. The Griffiths Report recommended the introduction of general management across the NHS and this precipitated the introduction of District and Unit General Managers within the recently formed District Health Authorities that replaced the abolished Area Health Authorities.

The establishment of the NHS in 1948 had sought to create a framework within which medical professionals could become salaried employees whilst retaining clinical freedom. The compromise that brought medical consultants into the NHS resulted in the application of the existing consultants' contract, and the arrangement whereby medical consultants employment contracts were held in the "remote filing cabinets" of Regional Hospital Boards (subsequently Regional Health Authorities). This was a clear signal to the medical profession that they were different from any other employee within the NHS, whose contract of employment was held at more local level. The culture created (at least in part) by this approach led to the comment in the recent Kennedy Report – following the enquiry into paediatric cardiac surgery at Bristol Royal Infirmary – that ...." Doctors always indicate that they have sessions at hospital X or that they attend clinic at hospital Y but they rarely admit that they are actually employed by hospital Z."...

The history and evolution of doctors in management is the continued attempt both at national and local level within the NHS to get doctors "on board" in the very real sense whereby they own and are accountable for the management of the resources which they commit. A financial budget arguably cannot be managed effectively unless it is managed by those who actually commit the resources. The continued failure of the NHS to deal effectively with this issue has resulted in many examples whereby medical consultants have a clinical power to commit resources but without the responsibility that must go with it to effectively manage those resources. Even today (some 20 years on from the birth of clinical directorates within the NHS) there are still clinical directorate budgets which are not "owned" by the clinicians who are spending them. This includes operating theatres and radiology in NHS Hospital Trusts and now Primary Care Trust commissioning budgets (given that General Practitioners spend separately from the PCT budget in practice).

The development of clinical directorates and (therefore) doctors in management in the early to mid-1980s was therefore stimulated by at least three issues – the recommendations for introducing general management throughout the NHS following the Griffiths Report; the outcome of the NHS Resource Management Initiative and its technique of specialty costing; and the use by the Government of the day of newly-available information to set activity and financial targets for the NHS.

The performance of the NHS started to be monitored by politicians and the media and the NHS fast became the "political football" that we witness today. It is interesting to reflect that the NHS was much less of a political football in the 1970s and early 1980s and indeed this reflected general acceptance by the main political parties that it was better to keep issues of funding and performance as "low politics" rather than "high politics" This, in turn, was related to the "deal" between the state and the medical profession whereby the former supplied resources (without political controversy) and the latter delivered the service (without much interference).

The availability of relatively good information within the NHS was a major stimulus in the evolution of doctors into management, both because it gave doctors the incentive of having resources to manage and use at local level (the power to commit resources became more balanced by the power to use resources more effectively), and because the Government of the day became far more vulnerable to criticisms both in the media, the public and other political parties regarding the performance of the NHS. This facilitated the setting of national and local targets for delivery, which is associated with a more interventionist approach in monitoring and managing performance. (It can be debated which came first!).

The evidence from recent NHS Medical Leadership Programmes (see Part 3 below) suggests that much of the "incentive" that was perceived in the 1990s for doctors to get involved in management (both at secondary and primary care levels) has actually diminished in some cases. The NHS has also witnessed the emergence of a new generation of newly-appointed NHS consultants who have different views from their predecessors – they are arguably more "corporate" when they reach consultant level (but not before), yet they clearly want to remain in control of their life outside of work. The stereotypical "old-style" consultants would expect autonomy but often give huge quantities of time and investment to the wider organisation (construed as the clinical community). Now, however, the plethora of national performance targets is clearly having a profound impact upon the continuing enthusiasm and ability of clinical directors and medical managers more generally within the NHS to deliver – to the extent where the annual round of commissioning and delivering through the Local Delivery Plan has perhaps become something of a treadmill. Medical leaders in secondary care seem almost "punch drunk" with the year-on-year demands for delivering cost improvements which have now been in existence for in excess of fifteen years.

For many GPs, the incentive to be "medical managers" has also diminished. Most GPs, do not wish to return to the inequitable policies and practices that flowed from GP Fundholding during the NHS internal market, yet the advent of Primary Care Trusts was intended to retain and develop the input of General Practitioners into the commissioning of services for their local health community. Yet the reality is that for the majority of GPs, this is not happening and commissioning is seen to be very much the preserve of a remote department at the centre of the PCT. It is possible that this an inevitable consequence of the natural evolution in the history of PCTs, given the agenda that they face and the timescale within which they were established.

The future wellbeing of the NHS is closely associated with a commitment by clinicians, and doctors in particular, to be at the heart of local management. The NHS must now "reinvent" the incentives for clinicians to be involved in leadership and management within the NHS. Crucial for the future is the reconciliation of the emerging Government policy of "patient choice" with appropriate clinical leadership and management responsibilities. The Patient Choice initiative needs to be worked-through extremely carefully if it is not at the same time both "re-empowering" and "dis-empowering". It might appear at this stage in its development to give more power back to the GP and/or the patient. This may remind us of various behaviours during the NHS internal market years when GP fundholders (armed with at least part of the Acute secondary care budget) only wanted to deal in commissioning terms with their secondary care clinical director counterparts. Yet the key difference is that the delivery of clinical services has changed quite fundamentally since the early 1990s, with the creation of clinical pathways and networks working *across* organisations and serving *wider* local health communities. This has stimulated managed clinical networks, thereby creating new clinical leadership and management roles.

Part 3 now outlines some of the specific issues addressed in medical leadership programmes.

PART 3: MEDICAL LEADERSHIP DEVELOPMENT

In November, 2001 the NHS Leadership Centre awarded the leadership development contract for both medical and clinical directors in secondary care to Keele University's Centre for Health Planning and Management. Working with its partners at Sheffield Hallam University, and the University of York, together with a panel of senior Trust Medical Directors and selected independent consultants, the Centre designed and delivered 24 leadership development courses between January, 2002 and March, 2003. 427 doctors attended these courses, of whom 141 were Medical Directors, 260 were Clinical Directors and 26 were Associate

Directors. In Spring, 2003 Keele was asked to extend its medical leadership portfolio. As a result, the 2003/2004 programmes will be offered to leaders in primary care and public health, as well as in the secondary sector and, increasingly to the wider clinical and managerial professions. It is anticipated that by March 2004, a further 620 participants will have had the opportunity to attend a leadership development course.

Aims and objectives; beliefs and values

It was clear that the fundamental aim of the programmes, from the viewpoint of the NHS Leadership Centre, was to create a nationwide cadre of medical and clinical directors capable of providing the leadership required to make a major contribution to the achievement of the overall aims and objectives of the NHS Plan and the "modernisation agenda". In other words, whilst the focus of the programmes was on developing individuals, the intended outcome was better organisational performance as a result of more effective medical leadership. Thus the development of individual medical leaders would lead to the development of the organisations within which they worked.

Some important beliefs (and values) about leadership and leadership development needed to inform both the design and the delivery of the programmes. Put simply, these were as follows:

i)   That, while there was no single overriding definition of leadership (and probably never could be) it was generally understood that leaders provided a sense of purpose and direction (for their team, organisation or country), could inspire, persuade and motivate people to follow them and had the skills to ensure that action resulted.

ii) That, equally, there was no single leadership style which was always effective – rather, an understanding of different approaches, and the circumstances in which they might be useful, was important for leaders.

iii) That to be personally effective, leaders nevertheless needed to develop and/or enhance certain attributes: ie

- Knowledge –of themselves and their own role, and of both the internal and external environments in which they operated.
- Creative abilities and skills – to understand their environment, to identify and articulate new opportunities and directions and to manage forward momentum.
- A set of appropriate qualities and behaviours (Garratt), to enable them to motivate and persuade others to think and act differently, and to sustain effort in periods of high activity or difficulty.

A combination of these elements gives credibility to a leader, without which he or she will be ineffective. These key elements of effective leadership were encapsulated in the "Keele Triangle", developed for the programmes and set out in Figure 2.1.

iv) That, fundamentally, development as a leader was a process of personal maturation which began with self-awareness and self-understanding and rapidly encompassed an ability to understand both the motives and behaviours of other people and the impact of one's own actions on others.

v) That this process of maturation needed to be taken at the speed of the individual, which would vary considerably, but which needed to encompass time for practice, and reflection on practice. The corollary

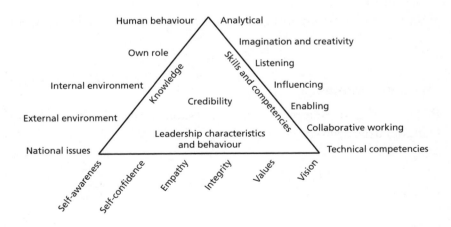

Figure 2.1: Effective leadership: the key elements

of this position therefore, for leadership programmes, was that, whilst short, intensive courses were important in focusing minds on the individual elements of the leadership "portfolio", it was also essential to offer ongoing support to enable a leader to reflect on his or her practice over time.

vi) That, finally, the successful design and delivery of leadership development programmes for doctors required a good understanding of this very particular audience, and appreciation of the level of intellectual exchange which must take place, in order to stimulate, challenge and energise a highly intelligent (but sometimes sceptical!) workforce.

The final overall objectives for the first two years of the medical leadership programmes, therefore, were to enable participants:
- To develop greater self-awareness, and self-knowledge, and to understand how personality affects preference for leadership style
- To develop their leadership capability by:
  - Understanding appropriate leadership styles and behaviours, using structured opportunities to reflect on their own, and others practice.
  - Acquiring greater knowledge of the wider policy agenda, allied to a deeper understanding of the role of the medical leader in the modern NHS.
  - Acquiring, or re-learning, some of the essential management skills, competencies and techniques which leaders need.
- To have personal support for the first six months of this development process.

The programmes

Boxes 1 to 5 give examples of the core sessions included in the five programmes delivered in years 1 and 2.

Box 1: Clinical directors

Core sessions
- Exploring individual personality and behaviour (using the Myers Briggs Type Indicator)
- Understanding leaders and leadership
- Understanding medical leadership and the Medical Directors' competency framework
- Exploring how to influence people and lead change
- Managing difficult situations
- Personal benchmarking and the preparation of personal development plans.

Box 2: Newly appointed Medical Directors

Core sessions
- Exploring personality and effective leadership (using the Myers Briggs Type Indicator)
- The Medical Director's role and competency framework
- Understanding the national policy agenda
- Understanding governance
- The challenges of change management
- Managing performance
- Personal benchmarking and the preparation of personal development plans.

Box 3: More experienced Medical Directors

Core sessions
- Understanding personality preferences and behaviour(using the Myers Briggs Type Indicator)
- Exploring the realities of the Medical Director's role: reflections on practice
- "So what sort of leader are you?": examining leadership style and effective leadership solutions
- Translating policy into practice: case studies from the NHS
- Managing conflict
- Exploring the dimensions of patient engagement
- Personal benchmarking and the preparation of personal development plans.

Box 4: Senior Medical Directors

Core sessions
- Inspirational leadership: exploring modern, effective, leadership practice
- "What about us?": exploring personal leadership styles and competencies
- The clinical leaders' challenge: managing improved performance
- The clinical leaders' dilemma: managing difficult colleagues
- "What do Medical Directors do next?": a discussion of future career options
- Visits to Department of Health, Downing Street, NICE/CHI to explore issues with national leaders
- "What about me?": 1-to-1 personal development planning sessions with tutors.

Box 5: Associate Medical Directors

Core Sessions
- Exploring individual personality and behaviour(using the Myers Briggs Type Indicator)
- Exploring leadership and leadership style
- Exploring the challenges of the Associate Medical Director role
- Understanding the national policy agenda
- Understanding governance
- Managing change and improving performance
- Handling conflict
- Creating and leading networks
- Personal benchmarking and the preparation of personal development plans.

Lessons learnt so far

All participants, on every course, were asked to evaluate the immediate impact of their programmes and the majority of participants on each course returned their forms. The analysis of this feedback for both years has given some interesting insights into both the preferred learning styles of senior medical staff, and the sessions which they cite as most useful for their personal development as leaders. In summary, the main findings were as follows:

Sessional content

- Whilst appreciating that some theoretical knowledge and understanding was important, medical leaders were keen to acquire practical skills on how to manage difficult or complex situations as leaders.
- In addition, participants wanted less policy analysis (they felt that they were reasonably knowledgeable in this field) and more practical tools about how to manage the dilemmas arising from the current NHS agenda.

Tutors and tutor groups

- The personal tutor role was considered to be of critical importance to the programmes. There were very favourable comments from almost all participants across both years. The tutors themselves very much enjoyed the role, but their experiences made them even more aware of the loneliness of the medical leader's position in the Service and the lack of support which many feel they are given by their own organisations.

Follow-up

- The original specification allowed for a one day follow-up and, for the first two years, it was decided that this should be three months after the initial residential module. In the first year, take up was variable, with sometimes as few as 35% of the original participants attending. In the second year, a higher percentage returned for the follow-up day and it was noted that it was important to fix the date for this event at the outset. Again, in an analysis of feedback from these one-day events, it was quickly noted that participants wanted more time working in small tutor groups and enjoyed the Action Learning concept in use.

The major programme elements eliciting the most favourable responses from participants were as follows:

- Personal tutor role
- Small group work
- Opportunities for networking

- The use of the Myers Briggs Type Indicator and the opportunity to explore personality and style
- The Medical Director's "toolkit", which was developed during the programme
- The sessions on managing change.
- The "handling conflict and managing difficult colleagues" sessions.

Key questions

There are a number of key questions arising from experience of the first two years' Medical Leadership Programmes. These questions raise issues directly for leadership development for doctors, but also indirectly for how the NHS is to be managed and indeed how health policy is to be implemented. The backdrop to all this is the relationship between doctors and the state, as outlined in Part I. This is not to deny the importance of local "corporate" management relationships (including medical leaders) within Trusts, but to point to the importance of the profession's self-perception and its relationship with Government.

i) Should medical leadership development be a uni-professional activity, or should all leadership development be conducted on a multi-professional basis? (There is also a different, supplementary question which is: do doctors learn best with their peers or with other professional groups?)

ii) At what point in a doctor's career should leadership development start and what are the appropriate staging posts?

iii) What is the most appropriate delivery point for effective medical leadership development – locally, when greater mutual understanding between colleagues, and creative partnerships with other professional groups, can be facilitated, or at a national level, when "stranger groups" offer a safer environment for mutual problem-sharing and, potentially, a richer diversity of experience for creative problem-solving?

iv) What are the most effective methods of development for medical leaders? For instance, are formal courses the most appropriate way to "kick-start" development, to be followed by other methods, such as mentoring or Action Learning sets, or are there other, more, or equally, effective methods?

v) Critically, what are we developing medical leaders to do? i.e. are we developing people who can motivate and lead a team within a hierarchical organisation, such as a secondary care Trust, or are we developing people who can work effectively in a managed clinical network or in a more informal partnership situation? Are the abilities and skills required similar or different?

Some of these questions, and most particularly those concerning multi-professional development and local programme delivery, are already being addressed by NHS Leadership Centre decisions on the future direction of development for doctors. Others remain the subject of considerable debate and/or require further research. What is certain, however, is that firstly, doctors' leadership development is of critical importance to the NHS if the ambitious aims of the NHS Plan are to be achieved, and secondly that the initial stages of such development need to start much earlier in the career ladder than is currently the case.

Conclusion

The challenge now is to forge a coherent link between the policy aspiration of "devolution and autonomy" with clinician self-management. This means exploring the links between existing acute Trust leadership and management and that of clinical networks; revisiting links between primary, secondary and tertiary care, and their management; providing coherent ownership of policy objectives and targets; clarifying the mix of centralism and local self-management; and reconciling patient choice with networked services.

The ideological component lies in transcending the rather sterile divide – sometimes synchronic, sometimes diachronic; sometimes descriptive, sometimes prescriptive – between hierarchies, markets and networks. Networks can be market-aiding or market-diminishing. In the NHS, patient choice within rationally-planned services should be the mantra, not markets.

Hard questions, however, remain. What will be the relationship between Trust Boards, Chief Executives and – for example – Medical Directors, on the one hand, and holistic, specialty-based clinical networks on the other? How will "lead Trusts" lead? How will doctor-managed networks avoid either the marketplace's or the state's embrace; and, if they stay self-managing, how will they manage performance to the satisfaction of the paymaster – Government, on behalf of the public – as well as local managers and the public? How will commissioning have to be re-shaped to prevent redundancy in a world of (let's be honest) provider-led planning, but in a modernised accountable form. These are but a flavour.

But the potential rewards are great. Again, just one example: a notable phenomenon of the current NHS is not just low medical morale but also low "top manager" morale. (Application rates for the best-paid and largest-Trust Chief Executive posts are one simple signal!) One of the reasons is high turnover; and the reason for this may well be increasingly structural. Chief Executives and Executive Directors are middle-men between Government and the medical profession rather than general managers. "All careers end in failure, eventually"....and now, usually sooner. The reason for this shortened cycle is the nature of targets, accountability and politicians' media-driven approach, on the one hand, and the medical profession's shortened patience with each new cycle of initiatives, in the current way of doing things. This shortened patience leads to the "new face as the basis of the new start", which is required more and more often.

A new settlement is needed. The bad news is that it is intangible but crucial. The good news is that much of current policy is valuable, and a new settlement does not need vast reorganisation in the sense of new institutions so much as simplification and elucidation. It also, however, needs a shared mission, difficult to achieve when the mission statement has been so discredited.

The key is renewed trust between the Government and the medical profession. Areas of consensus can be developed and communicated. Where consensus is not possible, compromises should be transparent, and likewise communicated. This process is likely to mean compromise between legitimate political targets and clinical aspirations. Fewer targets overall; greater clinical accountability within Trusts for performance and outcomes; and explicitly-recognised redrawing of the "resources/autonomy" conundrum as discussed above.

References

Clegg, S. (1990) *Modern Organisations: Organisation Studies in the Postmodern World*, London, Sage.

Department of Health (2001) *Learning from Bristol: The Report of the Public Enquiry into Children's Heart Surgery at the Bristol Royal Infirmary: 1984–1995*, London, Stationery Office.

Department of Health (2000) *The NHS Plan. A Plan of Investment, a Plan for Reform.*

Feachem, R., Sekrhi, N. and White, K. (2002) "Getting more for the dollar: a comparison of the NHS with California: Kaiser Permanente", *British Medical Journal*, Vol. 324, 19 January, pp 135–141.

Garratt, R. (1995) *Learning to Lead: Developing your Organisation and Yourself*, London, Harper Collins.

Jaques, E. (ed.) (1978) *Health Services: Their Nature and Organization and the Role of Patients, Doctors, Nurses and the Complementary Professions*, London, Heinemann.

Jessop, B (2000) *The Future of the Capitalist State*, Cambridge, Polity.

O'Connor, S. (1973) *The Fiscal Crisis of the State,* New York, Martin Robertson.

Moran, M. (1999) *Governing the Health Care State,* Manchester, Manchester University Press.

Paton, C. (2000) *World Class Britain: Political Economics, Political Theory and British Politics*, London, Macmillan.

CHAPTER THREE

Doctors in difficulty: leadership and performance

Sheila Peskett and Jennifer King

> "Leadership is not domination, but the art of persuading people to work towards a common goal"
>
> Goleman, 1996

In recent decades good leadership has come to be seen less in terms of instruction-giving and control and more as facilitating the release of energy and creativity of the led – transformational leadership. It is also recognised that leadership happens not just at the top of organisations but at every level, as organisational ambitions are taken forward by small teams sharing a vision.

Initial indications from the experience of dealing with doctors in whom there are concerns about their performance suggest that this is not being played-out as well as it might in the NHS. Doctors who find themselves in difficulty are usually highly-motivated and committed people but appear to be at odds with their organisations and colleagues. Individually, they lack leadership and team-working skills. They are unsure of what is expected of them and give mixed messages to people working with them about what they expect, particularly within the clinical teams that they should lead. We suggest, however, that there may also be a leadership deficit generally in their organisations, which have not recognised the needs and problems of these doctors and have not addressed them at an early stage in order to prevent poor performance and to improve patient care.

What has emerged in the evaluation of our work in this arena is an apparent clash of values between the doctors and the organisations in which they work. At times of stress, people and organisations may cling harder to their core values, thus exacerbating the rift. Values are guiding principles and when team members share similar values, team relationships usually work well and morale is high (West *et al.*, 2002). This seems to be far from the case when doctors are perceived to be difficult or when their performance is questioned.

Leadership defines the purpose or vision of an organisation or team with the values acting as the guiding principles to progress the way forward. The leadership at the top of the organisation should clearly articulate its vision and values and ensure that these are shared by the workforce. Values, however, should not only be stated but should be obvious and lived-out. There is evidence that where this happens in the commercial sector enhanced performance results (Collins and Porras, 1996). O'Reilly and Pfeffer (2000) stress the importance of aligning all internal processes with values and making these explicit. Companies that strive to do this and to resolve clashes of values build trust, motivation and commitment. So far the evidence is not available to show that this is happening in the NHS. Medical organisations rarely declare their values overtly, which can leave members unclear about what the organisation stands for (Pendleton and King, 2002). Although values tend to abound in medical bodies, it is often the standards that are emphasised. Both are powerful but it is values that state what is important and which tend not to vary. Standards state what is good or acceptable, which may well change in response to a number of factors. It would seem that it is more important for an organisation to know what it stands for than for where it is going.

Why are medical organisations reluctant to admit the importance of explicit shared values? Is it the adherence to standards? Is it because of a mistaken assumption that if every doctor behaves professionally, there will be organisational coherence? Or is there an almost irreconcilable difference among key stakeholders in the NHS, particularly doctors and managers, about the values they espouse that has made this too difficult to tackle? (Hunter, 2002). We are led to speculate that these dilemmas might underlie the reasons why organisations have found it difficult to resolve performance issues of some of their staff. We suggest that the issues of leadership and values and their inter-relationship need to be addressed more explicitly by organisations if they wish to improve individual performance and patient care.

Furthermore, part of leadership is establishing a positive work climate in order to create the conditions for people to give of their best. There is evidence that productivity can be powerfully affected by several psychological factors that together contribute to a positive working climate (Brown and Leigh, 1996). These include being clear about what is expected; being supported by management; being recognised for individual contribution and feeling free to challenge the status quo. This is further supported in the health sector by the work of West and colleagues (West, 2002) that shows clearly that effective feedback on performance and clarity about objectives are not only fundamental components of appraisal but also that feedback is associated with improvements in performance and reduction in error rates across all employment sectors. Training, or continued professional development (CPD), is also important in improving performance. Further, West *et al.* (2002) found a strong negative association between such people-management practices and patient mortality. The greater and the more sophisticated the levels of appraisal across all staff groups, the lower the patient mortality. This is probably linked to good team working, which in a wide variety of healthcare settings has been shown to predict quality of patient care (Borrill *et al.*, 2000) but is something that was almost always absent in our doctors undergoing assessment. The General Medical Council (GMC) stresses the importance of team-working by doctors but medical education and training until relatively recently has concentrated on individual achievement. Good team-working applies not only to clinical members but should include managerial and support staff and should engender a corporate commitment by everyone.

Most NHS organisations have mission statements, often collectively developed, that are committed to high-quality, patient-focused care and embrace the concept of valuing staff, but there is not always a sense that these are shared or openly enacted at all levels. The need for executives and managers to meet externally imposed targets does not always sit easily with professionals who have their own values and standards to follow. This 'ethos gap' (Fletcher, 1999) can only be bridged by high-calibre leadership at clinical and managerial levels. Openness, honesty and sharing of vision and values become of paramount importance. Instead what exists in many organisations is a climate of blame. This has led to an increasing level of alienation among doctors and these 'toxic emotions' (Frost, 2003) have serious adverse effects on performance and morale.

The situation, of course, is often even more complex in that people are usually working in healthcare systems involving more than one organisation, as expounded by Margaret Attwood and her colleagues in *Leading Change: A Guide to Whole Systems Working* (2003). Leadership is one of their five keys to whole systems development, with public learning, diversity, meeting differently and follow-through being the others. Values have to be shared across a wide range of bodies and professions to ensure effective change in improving patient care. Leadership is needed to keep the big picture in view and to provide the "holding framework" for the organisation's purpose and the people that work within it.

Doctors have usually entered medicine to care for patients. Their values are concerned with maintaining high standards of care and with doing the best for the individual patient in front of them. These have to be reconciled with a responsibility to use resources wisely and most effectively for the improvement of the health of the population as a whole. When there is intolerable tension between these two duties, or when doctors perceive that their managers or colleagues pursue an agenda of waiting list targets or balance sheets, doctors hold faster than ever to their professional values and may come to be thought of as behaving badly.

There have been some important steps forward in the last two years in tackling the issues of poor performance. There has been a recognition that the Medical Director in acute hospital services and equivalents in primary care, have a very significant role in helping to ensure that doctors share the organisation's aims and values; that they have clear and appropriate personal objectives; that they are properly trained and equipped for their jobs and that they have effective and motivating feedback. The NHS Leadership Centre's Medical Leadership Development Programmes have endeavoured to define the competencies needed by Medical Directors (Empey, Peskett and Lees, 2002). Developing individual performance and potential and developing team and corporate working are two of these competencies and both are highly relevant when trying to prevent poor performance.

The National Clinical Assessment Authority (NCAA), a special health authority established on 1 April 2001, following recommendations made in the Chief Medical Officer's report *Supporting Doctors, Protecting*

Patients (November, 1999) and *Assuring the Quality of Medical Practice: Implementing Supporting Doctors, Protecting Patients* (January, 2001). Providing a service to the NHS in England and Wales, the Prison Health Service and the Defence Medical Services, it supports organisations when they are faced with concerns about the performance of individual doctors or dentists.

The General Medical Council's (GMC) has developed standards of good medical practice against which doctors' performance should be assessed. They are:

- Good clinical care
- Maintaining good medical practice
- Relationships with colleagues
- Relationships with patients
- Teaching and training
- Probity
- Health

The principles of duties of a doctor, as defined by the GMC, underpin the values that doctors are expected to hold and espouse:

- Make the care of your patient your first concern
- Treat every patient politely and considerately
- Respect patients' dignity and privacy
- Listen to patients and respect their views
- Give patients information in a way they can understand
- Respect the rights of patients to be fully involved in decisions about their care
- Keep your professional knowledge and skills up to date
- Recognise the limits of your professional competence
- Be honest and trustworthy
- Respect and protect confidential information
- Make sure that your personal beliefs do not prejudice your patients' care
- Act quickly to protect patients from risk if you have good reason to believe that you or a colleague may not be fit to practise
- Avoid abusing your position as a doctor
- Work with colleagues in the ways that best serve patients' interests.

It is clear that there are many circumstances which could arise where a doctor may feel that a patient or patients may be at risk because of management action or directives. How these issues are handled is critical to the effective working and successful relationships of a doctor in the organisation. Good leadership skills on both sides are essential for this. Firth-Cozens and Mowbray (2001) review evidence to show how the personality and behaviour of leaders affects quality of patient care, including safety.

Research suggests (Cooke and Hutchinson, 2001) that core values of ensuring competency, the benefits to patient care of teamwork, skill mix and the use of clinical guidelines continue to be held by young doctors throughout their training, although there is considerable heterogeneity of the profession with multiple influences of personal characteristics, specialty socialisation and broader social changes shaping doctors' attitudes. How to ensure that these highly desirable values are maintained and nurtured is a test of leadership.

Personal qualities that influence behaviour include motivation, work style and values, interpersonal skills and relationships, emotional resilience, decision-making and judgement and leadership and influencing style – all of which should be taken into consideration when trying to help individuals and organisations deal with difficult situations or perceived value clashes.

Although the evidence base is still comparatively small, in our experience certain distinct typological patterns are emerging which should be noted and to some extent, perhaps, reflect the dissociation between professional and managerial groups. We have found that doctors in difficulty are usually people with very high and uncompromising standards who put pressure on themselves and others. Their love of new ideas and unconventionality is compromised by their poor self-discipline and high distractibility. They have difficulty in saying "No" and take on too much, being anxious to please. They tend to be altruistic and trusting and can then feel let-down and resentful when others do not live up to their expectations. They also have a high need for approval and are sensitive to rejection. They have low assertiveness and are not skilled in influencing or negotiating. Being anxious to get details right and avoid making mistakes, they are cautious decision-makers. They are inflexible when faced with uncertainty and have difficulty in coping with lack of structure and order in the work environment which leads to stress and adds to their poor personal organisation. Most significantly, perhaps, is that they tend to have an antagonistic style, not exploring alternative viewpoints and not valuing the contribution of others. This is combined with a lack of self-awareness and of the impact they have on others. They are not attuned to the emotional aspects of situations, often being task-focused and so are seen as insensitive. They convey mixed messages around leadership, wanting to take charge but also wanting to check-out decisions, thus conveying indecisiveness.

Primary care doctors often have a strong need for autonomy and are de-motivated with routine administration. They have a preference for a high degree of involvement with patients, sometimes over-extending themselves in putting patients first. They also, however, exhibit inflexibility, a tendency to get bogged down in detail and missing the bigger picture.

We have noted that almost all the doctors in difficulty demonstrate a lack of emotional intelligence – that ability to apply the right emotion or reaction, to the right degree, to the right person, at the right time, in the right way and for the right purpose (Goleman, 1996).

Our common diagnostic patterns can be summarised:

- Clash of values with management
- Distractions of varying nature leading to stress – personal problems, lack of facilities, poor team dynamics, isolated etc
- A "feedback vacuum" particularly in consulting or leadership skills, their lack of insight and their performance
- Lack of clarity about what is expected such as in their approaches to work, the culture of audit and professional development
- No training in leadership or influencing, team management, handling interpersonal conflict, learning styles
- Over-motivation leading to overwork and an inability to delegate
- De-motivation due to feeling under-valued, or from a chaotic environment
- Difficulty in thinking strategically, laterally or long-term
- Lack of training – treatment pathways, audit methods, basic research skills
- Playing safe so as not to take responsibility for a decision.

Leadership qualities are essential for effective working relationships and are closely linked to team-working skills. They are not confined to those in specific leadership roles, although senior doctors do, of course, have responsibilities for leading their clinical teams. As highlighted in Pakora *et al.*'s chapter, good leaders understand themselves, they develop the ability to understand the behaviour of others and, clinically, to build effective working relationships. In our experience, doctors in difficulty often lack this insight and ability. They become isolated and no longer have the benefits of peer or team support. We have probably failed to recognise and under-estimated the importance of leadership skills in every doctor at every level and the need to help them develop these attributes.

Leadership skills are not always inherent. They can be learnt like any others, although some people might have more natural talent, but they need to be developed, nurtured and practised. Much has been written on leadership theory with a growing recognition that not only is flexibility of style and approach needed by an individual but also that there needs to be a leadership culture and "mind-set" within an organisation to enhance good team working and deliver high quality patient care. Unfortunately, the development of leadership qualities has come relatively late to the NHS and to doctors in particular. Doctors in difficulty had been given little opportunity to develop their leadership potential. Moreover, they were often working in a feedback vacuum with no clarity abut what was expected of them. Few had had realistic objective-setting when appointed or thereafter and some had had no appraisal. Job descriptions were sometimes vague, giving no clear indication of what was expected or agreed, and induction often very superficial. This seems to demonstrate a lack of leadership on the part of the organisation as well as the doctors themselves.

Performance is influenced by many factors. Prevention always being better than cure, those factors that we can address we should do so. It seems that the first is to bridge the ethos gap (Fletcher, 1999) and tribal tensions between managerial and professional values (Hunter, 2002) to ensure that NHS values are explicit and embedded in the culture of all who work within the Service. The organisation's goals should be worked out openly and inclusively and individual and team objectives aligned to these. Feedback that is supportive, objective and positive rather than personally critical is essential and people should be made fit for purpose through adequate training and development. All this requires leadership not only at executive level but also at clinician level. There is a responsibility for all – organisations, employers, educators and individuals – to ensure that everyone is valued, and a recognition that all have a leadership contribution to improve patient care.

Successful organisations have explicit values and objectives and effective leadership. Leadership skills are needed at all levels. Our experience suggests that under-performers commonly lack these skills so upward and downward relationships suffer. It is hard, however, to exercise leadership in an organisation without explicit values and where organisational goals may not be understood. The NHS has some way to go before its leaders are primarily facilitators rather than instruction-givers and before its value systems and expectations are open and clear. If managers were more aware of the importance of leadership skills and the need to give feedback and offer training to potential under-performers, many unhappy, and sometimes tragic, circumstances might be avoided.

References

Attwood, M., Pedler, M., Pritchard, S., Wilkinson, D. (2003) *Leading Change: A Guide to Whole Systems Working,* Bristol, The Policy Press.

Borrill, C., West, M.A., Shapiro, D., Rees, A. (2000) "Team working and effectiveness in healthcare", *British Journal of Healthcare* Vol. 6, pp 364–371.

Brown, S . & Leigh, T. (1996) "A new look at psychological climate and its relationship to job involvement, effort and performance". *Journal of Applied Psychology,* Vol. 81, No 4, pp 358–368.

Collins, J. & Porras, J. (1996) "Building your company's vision", *Harvard Business Review,* Sep–Oct, pp 65–77.

Cooke, L. & Hutchinson, M. (2001) "Doctors' professional values: results from a cohort study of United Kingdom medical graduates", *Medical Education* Vol. 35, No, 8, pp 735–742.

Department of Health (1999) *Supporting Doctors, Protecting Patients,* London, The Stationery Office.

Department of Health (2001) *Assuring the Quality of Medical Practice: Implementing Supporting Doctors, Protecting Patients,* London, The Stationery Office.

Empey, D., Peskett, S. & Lees, P. (2002) "Medical leadership", *BMJ Careers ,* Vol. 325, No. 7376, pp 191–192.

Firth-Cozens, J. & Mowbray, D. (2001) "Leadership and the quality of care", *Quality in Health Care,* Vol. 10 (Suppl. II) pp ii3–ii7.

Fletcher, C., (1999) *Appraisal,* London, Institute of Personnel Management.

Frost, P. (2003) *Toxic Emotions at Work,* Harvard, Harvard Business School Press.

General Medical Council (2001) *Good Medical Practice*, 3rd edition, London, GMC.

Goleman, D. (1996) *Emotional Intelligence,* London, Bloomsbury Publishing Ltd.

Hunter, D.J. (2002) "A tale of two tribes: the tension between managerial and professional values", in New, B. & Neuberger, J. *Hidden Assets: Values and Decision-Making in the NHS,* London, King's Fund.

O'Reilly, C. & Pfeffer, J. (2000) *Hidden Power*, Harvard, Harvard Business School Press.

Pendleton, D. & King, J. (2002) "Values and Leadership", *British Medical Journal,* Vol. 325, No. 7376, pp 1352–1355.

West, M.A. (2002) "How can good performance among doctors be maintained?", *British Medical Journal Editorial,* Vol. 325, No. 7366, pp 669–670.

West, M., Borrill, C., Dawson, J., Scully, J., Carter, M., Anelay, S., Patterson, M. & Waring, J. (2002) "The link between the management of employees and patient mortality in acute hospitals", *International Journal of Human Resource Management,* Vol. 13, No. 8, pp 1299–1310.

CHAPTER FOUR

Clinical nursing leadership

Mike Cook

Whilst the need for effective clinical leaders in healthcare has been emphasised for several years, the term remains vague and bound up with the image of the lone "superhero" rather than an approach that draws on different strengths from different people at different times with a variety of clinical expertise. This chapter explores the definition of a clinical leader and introduces some of the research undertaken to find out more about the role, with a specific focus on nursing.

Definitions of leadership

Bryman (1999) suggests that there are three common elements in most definitions of leadership – influence, groups and goals. In other words leadership involves influencing other people, usually in some sort of group or team, to work towards an achievement of the group's goal. Earlier work by the author of this chapter (Cook, 1999) reflects this view in that an effective clinical leader is "an expert involved in providing or supporting direct care services, who influences others to continuously improve the care they provide".

Within the medical literature, Pendleton and King (2002) describe leadership in the following terms:

> "Leadership begins by defining a purpose: a compelling future that we are all trying to create and the values that will guide our actions along the way. Leadership re-examines the procedures that organisations follow and ensures that these procedures fully reflect the organisation's vision and values that they prepare it for its future challenges, rather than merely reflect its former glories. On these bases it builds an aligned community of like-minded and committed individuals who encourage one another towards their aims. Leadership inspires and then focuses effort so that motivation is not dissipated wastefully.

Leaders help organisations to articulate their values and make the tough choices needed to put the values into practice."

These definitions fit with the emergent view of clinical governance as "a framework through which NHS organisations are accountable for continuously improving the quality of their services and safeguarding high standards of care by creating an environment in which excellence in quality of care will flourish" (DoH, 1998). This definition is more complex than it first appears and is worth considering in more detail. The definition can be split into two parts. The first part emphasises accountability and continuous improvement, while the second emphasises the role of the leader, and has a much wider, and possibly more challenging, implication. To achieve an environment in which excellence in quality of care will flourish is a complex undertaking, requiring significant effort on the part of leaders in organisations.

These definitions highlight the complexity of the leader's role. They outline that an effective leader needs certain characteristics; certain competencies and an understanding of the impact of the environment on their effectiveness.

Why are effective clinical leaders important in today's healthcare settings?

Within the literature there has been general agreement that effective leadership is required to achieve high quality care. (Booth, 1995; Rowden, 1995; Maggs, 1996; Connolly, 1997; Smith, 1997; Salvage, 1999; Cunningham and Kitson 2000a,b). The context and policy drivers for these developments have been described in more detail elsewhere (see, for example, Cook, 2004). In summary, commitments have been made to modernise the health and social care sectors. *The NHS Plan* (DoH 2000a) commits the NHS to delivering a radical change programme which requires first-class leaders at all levels who should be "the brightest and the best of public sector management". The national nursing, midwifery and health visiting strategy for the NHS in England – *Making A Difference* (DoH, 1999a) stated "the Government's modernisation programme means that more nurses...need better leadership skills". *Meeting The Challenge: A Strategy For The Allied Health Professions* (DoH 2000b) promotes the leadership imperative for allied health professionals.

Modernising Health And Social Services: Developing The Workforce (DoH, 1999b*)* and *Service Quality Improvements In Social Care* (DoH 2000c) identify that excellent professional leadership and management capability enhance care provision.

This call for improved leadership is not restricted to the United Kingdom. Contacts with colleagues and groups across the world indicate that the importance of leadership in healthcare is recognized globally. The literature in the United States and Australia highlights this trend. The work of Burns (1978) and the theory of transformational leadership has been cited frequently in the American literature. This was emphasised by Marriner-Tomey (1993) an American nurse. She argued that the key to the development of nursing was transformational leadership: "The focus is upon change from a traditional hierarchical structure to one that pro- motes an entrepreneurial spirit through transformational leadership." (Marriner-Tomey,1993). Other American authors have also identified the importance of transformational leadership in achieving improvements in care (e.g. Loeffler, 1994; Sieloff, 1996; Kerfoot, 1997; Triolo *et al.*, 1997). Other research work in the USA identifies that investment in staff results in improved patient care and higher staff satisfaction (Aiken *et al.*, 2000).

An Australian nurse (Legg, 1996) identifies that an emergent Australian theme was that leaders in nursing were taking charge of areas that directly influenced and enhanced patient care. Legg described how nurse leaders led and managed the national case mix and case manage- ment agenda and stated that this was leading to positive outcomes for patient care, reduced length of stay and enhanced multidisciplinary care.

Research evidence

In the UK Newchurch & Co. and the NHS Executive (1995) published a report *"Sharpening The Focus: The Roles And Perceptions Of Nursing In NHS Trusts"*. The report highlighted the following about nurse leadership:

1. Career pathways were no longer obvious, and Trusts needed to facili- tate the process of development.

2. Exposure to strategic development needed to be included at an early career stage to allow development of the concept of the "bigger" picture.
3. Those nurses who had the required qualities and abilities must be identified early in their careers and given every encouragement to acquire the necessary skills and experiences to prepare them for their future career pathways which might be clinical, managerial or academic.
4. Nurses needed to be given the opportunity to gain new skills through shadowing, mentoring and networking with others both within and outside of their Trust. Exposure to different career experiences allowed nurses to obtain and develop a clear corporate view.

Part of this work reported an extensive international literature review of nursing leadership and despite an extensive search there was a paucity of research evidence and the review identified largely anecdotal and descriptive material.

From 1995, studies in clinical leadership have begun to emerge. Between 1997 and 2002 six empirical studies relating to clinical nursing leadership have been reported in the literature, (Kesington-Oloye, 2003). These studies are now summarised.

Antrobus and Kitson (1999) examined the broader social-political factors impacting on nursing leadership. The aim of the study was to examine critically contemporary nursing leadership within the context of health policy. Four research questions were explored:

1. What is the profile of nursing leaders who are considered to be effective in their leadership role?
2. How do leaders position themselves in relation to influencing in political, executive academic and clinical capacity?
3. What knowledge base and skills set can be identified for influencing in each of these domains?
4. How do leaders operate to influence the context within which they are working?

The sample consisted of 24 leaders who were recognised by their peers for their effectiveness in leading nursing. The findings of the study question the political success which the internally-focused nature of leadership has had for the profession. Nursing (and therefore nursing leadership) is shaped dramatically by the impact of politics and policy. The research discovered that in recognition of this, contemporary nursing leadership has both an internal and an external focus. Antrobus and Kitson identified that effective nurse leaders translated nursing into the language and priorities of politics, academia or management. The purpose of this translation was aimed at moving nursing from the invisible to the visible, so that in the translation the ideology and values of nursing were not lost, whilst nursing was positioned within mainstream thinking so that it acquired power and influence. They state that that, "effective nursing leadership currently is a vehicle through which both nursing practice and health policy can be influenced and shaped". (Antrobus and Kitson 1999). The following quotation from their work supported the importance of undertaking further research into clinical leadership:

> "Clinical leadership analysis is the most poorly-developed, reflecting perhaps a lack of investment in clinical practice and the lack of recognisable clinical leaders."

Hurst (1997) examined the leadership literature and reinforced this point, stating that the critical analysis of the theory and practice of nursing leadership was poorly-developed.

In 1998, Christian and Norman identified that clinical leadership was a key to developing nursing practice. The study explored how 28 Department of Health (DoH)-funded Nursing Development Units (NDUs) helped clinical leaders to develop. The study was part of a comprehensive evaluation of 28 DoH-funded NDUs to assess their "value-added" aspect so as to guide future policy developments in nursing and healthcare (DoH, 1993). The Department of Health wanted to encourage nursing-led initiatives through effective nursing leadership. One of the criteria required for the units to achieve NDU status, was to have an identified leader with day-to-day responsibility for the nursing care role. The respondents identified that the clinical leader was crucial in ensuring that the NDU operated to maximum benefit, and to maintain staff enthusiasm and confidence. The authors however, suggested that the position of the clinical leader within the organisational hierarchy was crucial in their effectiveness. To enhance the effectiveness of the clinical leader it was important to ensure that the role carried sufficient authority to engender change without the person being hampered by the operational management responsibility conventionally aligned to such roles.

Cameron and Masterson (2000)'s work Explored New Roles in Practice (ENRiP). Whilst focusing on Nurse Executives it also has relevance for clinical leadership, in that it identifies the difficulties and distractions faced by those that support clinical leaders. A qualitative study designed to explore the development of new professional roles, it looked at why these roles were developed and how professional groups led their development. They identified significant obstacles that faced Nurse Executives in exerting control over new role developments in their own Trusts, but in reality these challenges made an impact on all aspects of their work. The identified obstacles were:

- Organizational characteristics which mitigate against central planning and strategic development
- A lack of funding for service developments which generates a culture of reliance on charity
- Short-term government initiatives
- The imbalance of power between medicine and nursing at individual, organisational and policy levels
- The lack of coherent national policies and professional frameworks to assist Nurse Executives in leading health care development.

The authors stated that this environment led Nurse Executives to adopt a pragmatic approach to "muddling through". The Nurse Executive role itself is confounded by the manner of its implementation. Its success depends on personal relationships within the organisation and the existence of an executive commitment to professional leadership. Without such commitment many Nurse Executives find themselves with little control over the financing of nursing services or the professional agenda. The authors felt that the research explored views that up to that time had been largely ignored and concluded that the need for the role of Nurse Executive deserved attention from researchers and policy makers.

Cunningham and Kitson's (2000) explored the potential for an intensive 18-month educational programme – the Royal College of Nursing (RCN) Clinical Leadership Development Programme – to improve the leadership capability of ward sisters and senior nurses. The programme was based on a recognised link between effective clinical leadership and improved patient-centred care. The primary research question was whether the intervention improved the clinical leadership skills of participants. The programme emphasised a transformational leadership style as most appropriate for clinical nursing, as it was felt to promote a more participatory and emancipatory approach to leadership, promoting creativity, flexibility and speed of response, as well as accommodating personal development with more conventional leadership traits, such as the use of power, authority, influence and charisma. The focus of the programme was practical, experiential and work-based with an emphasis not just on skills acquisition but on an exploration of the attitudes, values and behaviours needed to produce leaders. A wide range of educational interventions were used with participants from a variety of different care settings. Participants were exposed to different role models and a spectrum of care experiences.

Twenty-eight nurse leaders were involved in the programme that was evaluated. Four were senior nurses and 24 were ward sisters. A range of tools were used to undertake the research, including:

- *Multifactor Leadership Questionnaire* (Bass, 1990): This tool explores 12 dimensions of leadership and predicts the leadership style of the respondent across a continuum from transactional to transformational. This was completed by the participants and their followers.
- *Organisation of Care* (Bowman and Thomson, 1995): This tool measures the way that nursing is organised and detects movement towards a more patient-centred care approach.
- *Newcastle Satisfaction With Nursing Scale* (McColl *et al.*, 1996): This tool measures the satisfaction reported by patients of the care provided by nurses.
- *Interdisciplinary Team Questionnaire* (Poulton and West, 1993): This tool explores the effectiveness of team working.

Other tools included "observations of care" where the participants were observed giving care on the ward and having their own area observed by an expert facilitator who had specific training for the observer role. "Patient stories" were also utilised and senior nurses and clinical leaders undertook and documented patient stories from the clinical area. A qualitative dimension was added through an analysis of the experiences of the programme participants.

The study's authors report that the research evidence supports the programme design. Findings indicate that the participants' leadership behaviour and nursing care changed towards a more patient-centred approach. A study undertaken by Cook *et al.* (2003) suggests that further research is required to investigate the long-term impact of the programme. The findings indicated that after completing a variety of leadership programmes, including the RCN programme, clinical leaders found it difficult to sustain the motivation required to continue the improvements started during the programme.

Manley's (2000) work focused on the interaction between the organisational culture and the consultant nurse, focusing on care outcomes. The study utilised an action research design in which a consultant nurse worked with and facilitated staff to achieve a new culture. The purpose of this study was to investigate the operationalisation of the role of the consultant nurse, for the purpose of providing better patient services. The work suggests that leadership should be recognised as the key to bringing about cultural change and acknowledges that a positive culture alone is insufficient. The work indicated that a nurse consultant with identified skills and ability would be extremely influential and likely to have a positive impact on the overall organisational culture and the performance of individuals and teams.

My own work has explored the attributes of effective clinical nurse leaders, Cook (2001a). The research focused on clinical leadership and identified five attributes of effective clinical leaders: *creativity, highlighting, influencing, respecting, and supporting.* Effective clinical leaders adopted a transformational leadership style and improved care, through others, by including transformational ("soft") knowledge as an integral part of their effective practice repertoire. Previous work explored nursing leadership through semi-structured interviews (Cook, 1999) and proposed that a combination of the leader's understanding and knowledge, values and beliefs, and cultural/organisational environment factors all contribute significantly to clinical nurses being effective leaders.

United States

In the USA published research demonstrates that effective leadership makes a difference to care outcomes. Aiken, Clarke & Sloane (2002) reported an international study of 10,319 nurses working in the United States, Canada, England and Scotland. They identified that dissatisfaction, burnout, and concerns about quality of care were common among hospital nurses in all five sites. Organisational/managerial support for nursing had a pronounced effect on nurse dissatisfaction and burnout and both organisational support for nursing and nurse staffing were directly, and independently, related to nurse-assessed quality of care. Multivariate results implied that nurse reports of low quality care were three times as likely in hospitals with low staffing and support for nurses as in hospitals with high staffing and support. The paper concluded that *"Adequate nurse staffing and organisational/managerial support for nursing are key to improving the quality of patient care, to diminishing nurse job dissatisfaction and burnout and, ultimately, to improving the nurse retention problem in hospital settings"*.

Laschinger *et al.* (1999) tested a model linking specific leader-empowering behaviours to staff nurse perceptions of workplace empowerment, occupational stress, and work effectiveness in a recently-merged Canadian acute care hospital. Leader-empowering behaviours significantly influenced employees' perceptions of formal and informal power and access to empowerment structures (information, support, resources, and opportunity). Higher perceived access to empowerment structures predicted lower levels of job tension and increased work effectiveness. Support for the model tested in the study highlighted the importance of nurse managers' leadership behaviours within healthcare organisations. Facilitative leadership styles were considered important to the success of work redesign efforts in hospital settings. In these work environments, staff members were empowered to make decisions based on their expert judgement and to act without seeking unnecessary permission from higher authorities. Lack of this kind of decision latitude has been linked to occupational stress and burnout among nurses.

Using Kouzes and Posner's (1993) model of leadership, McNeese-Smith (1996) found that staff nurses' perceptions of their managers' leadership behaviours were significantly related to their job satisfaction, productivity, and organisational commitment. Inspiring a shared vision was a significant predictor of organisational commitment, employee job satisfaction, and productivity. Kouzes and Posner (1993) argue that inspiring a shared vision is particularly important to such commitment during times of tension and change.

Other work from the USA identifies that effective leadership is also associated with excellence in care, this important link is made as part of the Magnet accreditation award (Balogh and Cook, 2003). This is also addressed in Houghton's chapter in this book.

Australia

Irurita (1992) and Morey (1996) indicated that nurse leaders were becoming more influential over health care policy. Astalos and Greenwood (2001) identify how effective clinical leaders working in Nursing Development Units were successful in improving both patient and staff satisfaction. They also cite a growing body of evidence that the stressors experienced by nurse leaders are threatening the survival of some of these units. The authors highlighted how the expectations and experiences of leaders changed over time with unanticipated pressures of work, a high turnover of clinical leaders, a perceived diminution of management support and unrealistic self-expectations. A significant theme that emerged as these stressors began to impinge was the leaders' own need for leadership support in order to sustain their confidence and motivation.

A study tour of Australia (Cook 2000) identified that whilst specific examples of effective practice amongst leaders was evident in Australia, the overriding impression was that Australia was similar to the UK and USA, namely that healthcare leadership varied from barely visible and ineffective to highly obvious and effective. It is suggested that this continuum will be the case internationally.

Three dominant themes are evident in the literature. These are – a call for leadership (UK-dominant), transformational leadership (USA-dominant) and advocacy for renaissance leadership (Australian-dominant). A theme common to the literature from all three countries was that leaders in nursing were important and that their abilities impacted directly on the standard of nursing care.

Views from other areas of the public sector in the UK

Within the UK, the Performance and Innovation Unit undertook a systematic study of leadership in the public sector (Cabinet Office, 2001). The report questions the idea that effective leadership provides the drive for change, and calls for more systematic work to explore this perceived "fact". The work highlighted that there was little shared understanding of the qualities required for effective leadership in today's public services and little evidence as to leader effectiveness. The report findings conflict with evidence cited earlier in this chapter and with evidence from the business sector where links between effective leadership and improved performance are made (Dahlgaard *et al.*. 1997, Joiner 1994). Additionally, the European Foundation for Quality Management (EFQM) excellence model has a central component of effective leadership. When the EFQM framework has been adopted, it has been shown to improve the quality of the business concerned, including healthcare (Stahr *et al.*, 2000).

The Cabinet Office study indicated that further investment was required to support research into effective preparation for leaders in the public sector and to explore how effective leadership impacted on the service provided. Despite this call for greater clarity, few if any resources have been made available for research or systematic study of what is or what should be an effective public sector leader.

School leadership has also been extensively examined over several years (see for example Sergiovanni, 1992; Thody 1997; West-Burnham 1997) and this has spawned several programmes for headteachers such as the Leadership Programme for Serving Headteachers (LPSH) (TTA, 1998) and the National Professional Qualification for Headship, (Collarbone, 2001). Both schemes strongly promote the "lone superhero" leader. For instance the LPSH scheme appears to pay no attention to the vital contribution made by heads of department to school improvement – which was comprehensively researched by Torrington and Weightman (1989) and Earley and Fletcher-Campbell (1989). These authors identified that effective leadership at *all* levels was important, but that department heads were seen as the driving-force behind any school. They highlighted that leadership qualities existed at all levels and releasing these would enhance further school improvements. Ogawa and Bossert (1995) reinforce this point, arguing that leadership should be associated with roles throughout an organisation, although the needs of leadership will change depending on the position in the organisation. This same point is made by Fidler (1997) where he writes "Although leadership from senior figures is important, many other positions and individuals in schools should be encouraged to provide leadership for particular tasks or sections of the school". Naturally this also has the benefit of preparing people for new leadership positions as they arise.

It is interesting that leaders in both healthcare and education speak of the need for freedom and how the ever-increasing demands from centralised policy makers (e.g. hospital waiting-times and pupil attainment targets) impact negatively on their work. Given the high degree of external control faced by leaders in the public sector, it is striking that the Cabinet Office state that "in most cases leaders need more freedom to lead ... Nonetheless, the number of cases is small in which detailed external control over process is justified, and it remains true that a key to promoting leadership is to allow leaders space to lead. Government must be sparing in the number of frameworks that it sets. Leaders who are overburdened with directions will be unable to function effectively."

Freedom to lead – one Trust's approach

A study undertaken between 2001 and 2003 explored the clinical leadership role of the ward sister/charge nurse at one teaching hospital NHS Trust in east London. The research was conducted with ward sisters and charge nurses working in ten different acute specialties and was designed to explore the impact of providing the G grade sisters and charge nurses with £16,000 each, to spend in ways which would support their clinical leadership capacity.

The G grade sisters and charge nurses had attended (or were attending) a variety of leadership development initiatives. The allocation of £16,000 represented the Trust's recognition that clinical leaders cannot be fully effective without adequate resources and support.

Data were collected through individual interviews, collages (pictorial representations of the G grades' views), diary records, group discussion and documentary analysis.

Overall the ward leaders viewed the clinical leadership development initiative positively, especially in terms of practice development and personal job satisfaction. Recruitment and retention of nursing staff was, however, regarded as a continuing problem. Ten recommendations emerged (Cook *et al.*, 2003) relating to:

- Recruitment, retention and succession planning
- Involvement in central decision-making
- An increased awareness of external policy drivers
- Continued investment in staff development
- Improvement in skills in prioritising
- An increased awareness of diversity issues
- Improved skills in complex cancer care (especially when care is provided in non-specialised settings)
- Ensuring that positive change strategies are utilised
- Encouragement of measured risk taking to develop and improve services
- Encouragement of time to explore the frustration factors experienced by the ward leaders.

It is suggested that staff in other Trusts would recognise these recommendations as useful for them to consider in their own areas.

Conclusion

This chapter has provided a brief overview of research into clinical leadership with an emphasis on clinical nurses. Further work is still required to gain deeper understanding about clinical leadership. Research into nursing leadership has started and whilst this requires more work, attention also needs to be focused on other healthcare professionals. A significant gap in the current knowledge is research that investigates what makes clinical leaders effective in terms of health outcomes. This needs to be of an inter-professional nature and needs to explore the impact of clinical leaders within the context of their working environment.

References.

Aiken, L., Clarke, S. and Sloane, D.(2002) "Hospital Staffing, Organisation, And Quality Of Care: Cross-National Findings". *International Journal For Quality In Health Care* Vol. 14, No. 9, pp 5–19

Aiken, L., Havens, D. & Sloane, D. (2000) "Magnet nursing services recognition programme", *Nursing Standard*, Vol. 14, No. 25, pp 41–47.

Antrobus, S. & Kitson, A. (1997) *Nursing Leadership in Context: A Discussion Document*, London, Royal College of Nursing.

Atsalos, C. & Greenwood, J. (2001) "The lived experience of clinical development unit (nursing) leadership in Western Sydney, Australia [experience before and throughout the nursing career]" *Journal of Advanced Nursing*, Vol. 34, No. 3, pp 408–416.

Balogh, R., Cook, M. & Smith, H. (2003) *Attracting Evidence for Magnet Accreditation: The First Experience of Attempting and Gaining Magnet Accreditation Outside the USA at Rochdale Healthcare NHS Trust, UK,* St Martin's College, University of Lancaster. Also http://www.city.ac.uk/barts/research/reports/pdf/cook_m/magnet%20.pdf.

Bass, B. (1990) *Bass and Stogdill's Handbook of Leadership Theory, Research and Managerial Application,* 3rd edition, London, Free Press.

Bryman, A. (1999) "Leadership in organisations" in Clegg, S., Hardy, C. & Nord, W. (eds), *Managing Organisations,* Thousand Oaks, Sage, pp 26–42.

Booth, B. (1995) "Leading frights ... effective leaders", *Nursing Times,* Vol. 91, No. 23, p. 58.

Bowman, G. & Thomson, D. (1995) *A Classification System for Nurses' Work Methods: The Bowman Classification,* Oxford, National Institute of Nursing.

Burns, J. (1978) *Leading Ability,* New York, Harper and Row.

Cabinet Office (2001) *Strengthening Leadership in the Public Sector: A Research Study,* Performance and Innovations Unit, London, Cabinet Office. Also: http://www.cabinet-office.gov.uk/innovation/leadershipreport/piu-leadership.pdf.

Cameron, A. & Masterson, A. (2000) "Managing the unmanageable?: nurse executive directors and new role developments in nursing", *Journal of Advanced Nursing,* Vol. 31, No. 5, pp 1081–1088.

Christian, S. & Norman, I. (1998) "Clinical leadership in nursing development units", *Journal of Advanced Nursing,* Vol. 27, No. 1, pp 108–116.

Collarbone, P. (2000) Aspirant heads, *Managing Schools To-day,* (June/July) pp. 28–31.

Connolly, M. (1997) "The naked truth....nursing leadership", *Nursing Times,* Vol. 93, No. 12, p. 27.

Cook, M.(2004) "Multi-professional post-qualifying education" in Glen, S. & Lebia, T. (eds.) *Team Leadership: Interprofessional Post Qualification Education for Nurses: Working Together in Health and Social Care*, London, Palgrave Macmillan.

Cook, M. (2001a) "The renaissance of clinical leadership", *International Nursing Review,* Vol. 48, pp 38–46.

Cook, M. (2001b) "The attributes of effective clinical leaders", *Nursing Standard (Art and Science)* Vol. 15, No. 35, pp 33–36.

Cook, M. (2000) *Clinical Leadership Skills in Australia,* Florence Nightingale Travel Scholarship, Report Of Scholarship Award.

Cook, M. (1999) "Improving care requires leadership in nursing", *Nurse Education Today,* Vol. 19, No. 4, pp 306–312.

Cook, M., Goreham, C.; Smith, H. & Young, G. (2003) *Supporting G Grade Leadership at the Homerton University Hospital NHS Trust: an Evaluation,* Internal Research Report, City University. Also: http://city.ac.uk/barts/research/reports/pdf/cook_m/homertonejb.pdf.

Cunningham, G. & Kitson, A. (2000) "An evaluation of the RCN Clinical Leadership Development Programme: Part 1", *Nursing Standard,* Vol. 15, No. 12, pp 34–37.

Cunningham, G. & Kitson, A. (2000) "An evaluation of the RCN Clinical Leadership Development Programme: Part 2", *Nursing Standard,* Vol. 15, No. 13, pp 34–40.

Dahlgaard, J, Larsen, H. & Norgaard, A. (1997) "Leadership profiles in quality management", *Total Quality Management,* Vol. 8 (2 & 3) pp 516–530.

Department of Health (1998) *Modernising the Health Services in London: A Strategic Review,* London, Department of Health.

Department of Health (1999a) *Making a Difference: Strengthening the Nursing, Midwifery and Health Visiting Contribution to Health and Healthcare,* London, Department of Health.

Department of Health (1999b) *Modernising Health and Social Services: Developing the Workforce,* London, Department of Health.

Department of Health (2000a) *The NHS Plan: A Plan for Investment: A Plan for Reform,* London, Department of Health.

Department of Health (2000b) *Meeting the Challenge: A Strategy for the Allied Health Professions,* London, Department of Health.

Department of Health (2000c) *Service Quality Improvements in Social Care,* London, Department of Health.

Earley, P. & Fletcher-Campbell, F. (1989) *The Time to Manage* London, National Foundation for Educational Research.

Fidler, B. (1997) "School leadership: some key issues" *School Leadership and Management,* Vol. 17, No. 1, pp. 23–37.

Hurst, K. (1997) *A Review of the Nursing Leadership Literature,* Nuffield Institute for Health, University of Leeds.

Irurita, V. (1992) "Transforming mediocrity to excellence: a challenge for nurse leaders", *Australian Journal of Advanced Nursing,* Vol. 9, No. 4, pp 15–25.

Joiner, B. (1994) *Fourth Generation Management: The New Business Consciousness,* New York, McGraw-Hill.

Kerfoot, K. (1997) "On leadership: leadership: believing in followers", *Dermatology Nursing*, Vol. 9, No. 3, pp 194–5.

Kesington-Oloye, R. (2003) *Literature Review: Making a Difference: Clinical Nurse Leadership?*, Unpublished BSc thesis, City University, London.

Kouzes, J. & Posner, B. (1993) *Credibility: How Leaders Gain and Lose it, Why People Demand it.* San Francisco: Jossey-Bass.

Laschinger, H., Wong, C., McMahon, L. & Kaufmann, C. (1999) "Leader behavior impact on staff nurse empowerment, job tension, and work effectiveness", *Journal of Nursing Administration*, Vol. 29, No. 5, pp 28–39.

Legg, S. (1996) "The learning profession in nursing: the leading edge of care", *Nursing Standard Supplement*, Vol. 10, No. 24.

Loeffler, S. (1994) "Leadership characteristics and change seeker need of nurse managers as predictors of readiness for a participatory nursing management model", *Kentucky Nurse*, Vol. 42, No. 3, p 23.

Maggs, C. (1996) "Debate: professors of nursing as clinicians and academics: is this the way forward?", *NT Research*, Vol. 1, No. 2, pp 157–158.

Manley, K. (2000) "Organisational culture and consultant nurse outcomes: Part 1: organisational culture", *Nursing Standard*, Vol. 14, No. 35, pp 34–38.

Marriner-Tomey, A. (1993) *Transformational Leadership in Nursing*, St Louis, Mosby.

McColl, E. (1996) "A study to determine patient satisfaction with nursing care", *Nursing Standard*, Vol. 10, No. 52, pp 34–38.

McNeese-Smith, D. (1996) "Increasing employee productivity, job satisfaction and organizational commitment", *Hospital and Health Service Administration*, Vol. 41, No. 2, pp:160–175.

Morey, W. (1996) "Student corner: total quality management and nursing: a shared vision", *Contemporary Nurse: A Journal for the Australian Nursing Profession*, Vol. 5, No. 3, pp 112–116.

Newchurch & Co./NHS Executive (1995) *Sharpening the Focus: The Roles and Perceptions of Nursing in NHS Trusts*, London, Newchurch & Co.

Ogawa., R. & Bossert, S. (1995) "Leadership as an organisational quality", *Educational Administration Quarterly* Vol. 31, No. 2 pp. 224–243.

Pendleton, D. & King, J. (2002) "Values and leadership", *British Medical Journal* Vol. 325, pp 1352–1355.

Poulton, B. & West, M. (1993) "Effective multidisciplinary teamwork in primary healthcare", *Journal of Advanced Nursing*, Vol. 18, No. 6, pp 918–925.

Rowden, R. (1995) "Crisis? What crisis?", *Nursing Times*, Vol. 91, No. 37, p. 50.

Salvage, J. (1999) "Speaking out … supersisters … clinical leadership", *Nursing Times*, Vol. 95, No. 21, p. 22.

Sergiovanni, T. (1992). *Moral Leadership: Getting to the Heart of School Improvement*, San Francisco, Jossey-Bass.

Sieloff, C. (1996) "Nursing leadership for a new century", *Seminars for Nurse Managers*, Vol 4, No. 4, pp 226–33.

Smith, S. (1997) "The loneliness of a long-term leader", *Nursing Times,* Vol. 93, No. 12, pp 30–31.

Stahr, H., Bulman, B. & Stead, M (2000) *The Excellence Model in the Health Sector: Sharing Good Practice*, Kingsham Press.

Teacher Training Agency (1998) *Leadership Programmes for Serving Head-Teachers: Handbook for Participants*, London, Teacher Training Agency.

Thody, A. (1997) *Leadership of Schools: Chief Executives in Education.* London, Capsules.

Torrington, D. & Weightman, J. (1989) *The Reality of School Management,* Oxford, Blackwell.

Triolo, P., Pozehl, B. & Mahaffey, T. (1997) "Development of leadership within the university and beyond: challenges to faculty and their development" *Journal of Professional Nursing*, Vol. 13, No. 3, pp 149–53.

West-Burnham, J. (1997) "Leadership for learning – re-engineering 'mind sets'." *School Leadership and Management,* Vol. 17, No. 2, pp 231–244.

CHAPTER FIVE

Leadership development and job effectiveness

Perceptions of clinicians who have undertaken a Master of Arts programme in leading innovation and change

Amanda Thomas

The NHS Plan (2000) aims to modernise the NHS, requiring delivery through effective leadership and management at all levels within the Service. How do we develop clinicians as leaders and managers? This chapter examines the influence of a Master of Arts programme in Leading Innovation and Change (MALIC) on a group of clinicians, exploring their perceptions of leadership development, career development, and job effectiveness after undertaking the MALIC.

At the time of writing this chapter, I had become an Associate Medical Director of a Community Children's Service and had recently transferred to a Primary Care Trust. My existing work pattern changed significantly and I became interested in the training needs of clinicians moving to similar roles.

Introduction

The National Health Service is the largest organisation in the UK, employing over one million people with a budget of £65.4 billion in 2002–2003, rising to an estimated £105.6 billion in 2007–2008. The founding principle of the NHS remains the same today as when it was created:

> "The NHS is a British ideal, free at the point of need for everyone in every part of Britain."
>
> Chancellor of the Exchequer Gordon Brown,
> Budget Speech, 2002

Since the early 1980s, a number of reforms have occurred, driven by the following factors:

- A dramatic growth in science and technology
- A parallel growth in the cost of healthcare
- Strong public support for the NHS to remain in the public sector
- Growing expectation of the service by the public
- Doubts about the appropriateness and value of existing patterns of clinical organisation
- Concerns over the medical profession's capacity to ensure accountability of its members following the *Bristol* and *Shipman Inquiries* (Davies and Harrison, 2002; Degeling *et al.*, 2002)

Reforms have occurred with increasing rapidity through three phases:

Phase 1: A service administered by multi-disciplinary management teams operating by consensus

Phase 2: A system based on private sector principles of general management, operating in an internal market for healthcare

Phase 3: A system comprising the above two with general management retained but operating within a framework of planning, collaboration and partnership.

Nationally-determined strategies and objectives, national programmes for quality, clinical effectiveness, research and development, and education and training have underpinned these changes. The most recent and far-reaching change followed the introduction of the NHS Plan (2000). *Delivering The NHS Plan* (2002) contains a package of reforms aimed at devolving the health service to frontline staff who will have greater flexibility and increased freedom to practice more effectively. Delivery of the NHS Plan requires structural and cultural changes, as set out in the Government document, *Shifting The Balance Of Power* (DoH, 2001), and effective leadership and management at all levels within the Service.

Since the *Griffiths Report* of 1984, the drive to involve clinicians in management has increased in impetus. Recognised advantages of involving doctors in management include:

- Control of expenditure through co-operation and active participation of doctors

- Decentralisation of the management decision-making process by delegating down to those responsible for delivering the service
- Improved communication from the Board to the frontline staff and vice-versa
- Bringing doctors on board within the organisation
- Breaking down barriers between professional groups and hierarchies
- Improved planning and clarity of service objectives.

(Walker and Morgan, 1996)

Tensions between management and medicine have always existed but there is a growing sense of urgency to harmonise this tension to facilitate the modernisation of the NHS. The introduction of the clinical directorate model attempted to involve doctors in management by creating a decentralised organisation with authority and responsibility devolved to doctors in each specialty or directorate. Clinicians were offered opportunities to be part-time managers as well as retaining their clinical role. For those who entered these roles new tensions were created – those of conflict between balancing the clinical and managerial roles and the lack of training for the roles.

Prior to the 1990s, management training for doctors was haphazard and sparse, and almost non-existent at medical undergraduate level (Walker and Morgan, 1996). In recognition of the need, the Department of Health funded limited management programmes for doctors between 1990 and 1993 and, following the Calman Report in 1993, the Calman training of Specialist Registrars included management training.

The emphasis on management training has now been switched to a focus on leadership development with the requirement of effective leadership to deliver the NHS Plan. The NHS Leadership Centre (as part of the NHS Modernisation Agency) was created to facilitate change and support leadership development of local staff. The MALIC course described in this chapter developed through collaboration between the Centre for Leadership and Management at the University of York and the School of Management Community, and Communications at the College of Ripon and York St. John. The aim of the course is:

> "To provide an opportunity for leaders of innovation and change to work together on issues which will have significant impact within their organisations."

The course aims to provide:

"A wide-ranging, informed and systematic approach to management and leadership so that both organisational and individual potential are enhanced. Participants will chose particular issues which they will identify for resolution and development within their own organisations. The course will provide frameworks and opportunities for supervised reflection, skill development and networking."

The objectives of the course are set out in Box 5.1.

Box 5.1: MALIC course objectives

1. Examine the contributions of various theoretical models and approaches to leadership, innovation and change within organisations
2. Explore the different facets of effective leadership
3. Assess personal and professional strengths and areas for development as leaders
4. Design and implement a research project relating to leading innovation and change within an organisation
5. Demonstrate leadership of innovation and change as part of strategic development in an organisation
6. Identify and evaluate culture in an organisation
7. Evaluate leadership styles appropriate to specific situations
8. Refer critically upon ethical dilemmas within the decision-making process in organisations
9. Systematically reflect upon learning, practice and experience.

There has been little evaluation research on leadership programmes in the NHS and there is little data on the effectiveness of current leadership programmes for clinicians.

The research

The aim of the study was to explore the influence of the MALIC on a group of clinicians that had undertaken the course. The "grounded theory" approach developed by Glaser and Strauss (cited in Denscombe, 1998 and Mason, 1996) was used, as illustrated in Figure 5.1, with no preconceived set of hypotheses or theories to test and aiming to explore the clinicians' experiences. Emerging concepts and theories were developed and refined during the process of the research and examined in

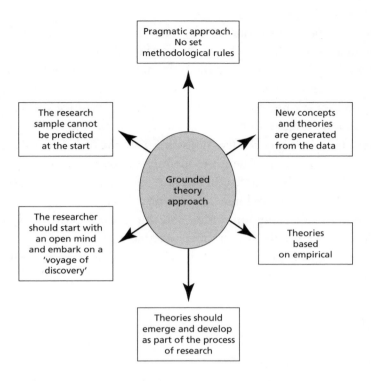

Figure 5.1: Grounded theory approach to analysing qualitative research

relation to current theory at the end of the process. Parry (cited in Gaughan 2001) argues that leadership is a *social influence process* and suggests the use of qualitative research methods for the study of leadership, highlighting the "grounded theory" approach as the most appropriate method.

Semi-structured, qualitative interviews were chosen to obtain more in-depth, rich data with the potential for a higher response rate than questionnaires. In the time available, Ten out of twelve clinicians were interviewed (seven males and three females), each of whom had achieved a MALIC with the College of Ripon and York St. John and the University of York since the programme's inception. The ten interviewees comprised of two Directors within Primary Care Trusts (PCTs), three Hospital Consultants, one Lead Clinician, two Clinical Directors, one Associate Medical Director and one Medical Director.

The interviews were one-to-one, semi-structured, taped and lasted approximately one hour. They were conducted informally and flexibly with twelve questions covering the influence of the MA on the interviewee's career development; the reasons for undertaking the course; their perceptions of themselves as leaders; the perceived positive benefits of the MA; common issues and dilemmas arising from formal leadership/management roles, and any changes occurring after the MA. Critical incident reports were used in an attempt to identify emergent managerial or leadership competencies that could support the clinicians' perceptions of their own leadership development. The interviewees were invited to bring two examples of leading innovation and change, which they had personally developed since the MA, to their interview.

The full transcripts were coded and patterns and themes emerging from the data were categorised.

Results

Job or role changes post MA

All ten clinicians had changed jobs or roles either during or after the MA course. Four clinicians perceived that the MA had influenced their decision to change their jobs or roles. Developing insight, an understanding of organisational culture, leadership and management, and an awareness of their own abilities and skills emerged as the influences from the course.

> "I think through the MA rightly or wrongly... I realised that I was as well-equipped as anybody."

NHS reforms involving the abolition of Health Authorities and the creation of PCTs forced two clinicians to apply for posts in new organisations. The support from the course tutors and participants were powerful influencing factors, as well as the skills developed from the course, for coping and managing the change process.

Four clinicians could not directly attribute any influence from the MA on their role change. All were experienced clinicians with some self-belief and self-awareness of their natural ability towards leadership.

Reasons for applying for the MA

Training, skill enhancement and personal development for formal management/leadership roles underpinned by an evidence base (theoretical knowledge), protected study time and time out, were themes emerging as more frequent reasons for applying to do a MALIC.

> "I was going to have to learn those skills and learn more about them anyway in order to be able to succeed in the Clinical Director role."

Other themes mentioned included networking, self-reflection and opportunity (through advertising by tutors, other participants, or mailing).

Current role

Leadership appeared to be more strongly emphasised as the role the clinicians were adopting either informally or formally after the MA.

> "So I was first professional, then manager, then I thought 'no, I've got to be honest, I do have a leadership responsibility."

Where clinicians were in a role with management responsibilities, there was still an emphasis towards leadership with some delegating almost all management duties or working in close partnerships with general managers.

> "Mostly a leadership role...because I got some very good operational managers who do most of the pure management work."

The reasons given for applying for formal roles were a combination of perceived natural aptitude in management/leadership coupled with role availability and in some cases a drive to lead or be in control.

Difficulties with formal roles emerged in the interviews of eight clinicians that were or had been in a formal management role. Conflict in time and in prioritising managerial and clinical work had led some clinicians to an imbalance in home/work commitments. Clinicians perceived that the reduction in clinical work, due to management work, had led to a loss of respect with colleagues and an inability to progress clinical skills. Clinicians also discussed difficulties establishing credibility with clinicians and managers both in a dual role of manager and clinician or where they were in a single role with no clinical workload. The role was described as unpopular, with no-one wanting to fill the post and no succession planning, having no real power, apart from persuasion, and being an un-elected position that was not representative causing conflict when having to implement changes or unpopular Trust Board decisions.

Influence of the MA on job effectiveness

The data were rich with the perceived positive benefits of undertaking the MA for the individual clinicians in their roles at work, the skills they have acquired to perform their roles and their personal development. All ten clinicians perceived the course to have had a positive influence on themselves or their ability to perform their roles more effectively. All of the clinicians perceived that the training in management/leadership from the course had a positive effect on their work from their ability to apply the theoretical knowledge from the course into practice (in terms of leading, managing and implementing change), applying their learning back to their organisations, training others in leadership and changing their attitude (more favourably) towards managers.

Most of the clinicians perceived positive effects from their acquired depth of knowledge of the theory of management, leadership and change regarding the course experience as 'always in the background', enabling them to understand structures and systems and change implementation. The continued use of course material for reference during their current work was also highlighted.

> "There is whole load of stuff you learnt during the MA and a lot of it was obviously very useful, but most of it you use subvertly not overtly. It is just there in the background, so that things spring to mind occasionally, so to actually have some theoretical depth of knowledge – the theoretical perceptive is quite important"

Skill acquisition was a common theme with nine clinicians perceiving increased confidence in themselves and credibility with Trust managers. Particular skills described included talking the same language as managers, being able to recognise strengths and weaknesses of others, valuing people, the development of people skills/managing people in other ways, and adopting a different approach or style to situations.

"You can talk the same language as they can. In the medical language there is clearly...there is also a management language and I think it gives you that advantage."

Eight clinicians perceived that they had personally developed in themselves or in areas of leadership, change management and career direction. Three clinicians appeared to be using the MA as a building block to continue self-developing as leaders (e.g. leadership development course).

The benefits of self-reflection emerged in seven interviews and included perceptions of a greater self-awareness or understanding or a greater awareness or understanding of other people. Seven clinicians described benefits from networking, categorised by meeting other people, learning from other people, learning from others experiences and receiving support from others.

"The MALIC was brilliant. I thought that the networking bit was really the very best part of it."

Three clinicians described the support from the course participants and tutors as essential to them during a period of considerable difficulty and change at work. Learning from other people was a recurrent theme. Clinicians found it helpful to hear others' experiences using modelling techniques, brainstorming, group thinking, problem solving and mutual support.

"I think it was often more useful to know what other people's experiences and the problems they were having and the approaches they have taken or whatever."

'Seizing opportunities' emerged as a theme from six interviews with clinicians seizing opportunities to take on new roles, further training programmes and using research techniques developed on the course.

Five clinicians perceived benefits from the opportunity to study academically and within this described the positives of having protected time, studying material appropriate to their needs, achieving a postgraduate qualification, undertaking research and using new research techniques.

"It was immensely helpful in having the time out once a month... Just the discipline of not being here for two days a month was wonderful...Just the space to actually think away from a work environment. it was extremely, extremely useful."

Two clinicians reported using the course tutors for training purposes within their own organisations, after the MA.

Leadership development

All ten clinicians perceived that they had developed as leaders following the MA. Their responses were categorised into two themes, the first included personal qualities that are commonly encountered in leadership (self-belief; self-awareness; a driver of innovation and change; humility and personal integrity-to include belief in their own personal values, their resilience and honesty) and the second included elements of how the clinicians perceived that they had developed as leaders since the MA.

Within the theme of personal qualities, all ten clinicians expressed greater self-awareness and knowledge of their strengths and weaknesses (a number of clinicians cited the leadership profiling as facilitating this process) also indicating there were opportunities to build on their strengths and gaps. Personal Integrity emerged in eight interviews with the interviewees exposing their values, demonstrating their fairness in approach to others and their respect for diversity.

"You need to persuade people to do things...that's leadership...you know...and you've got to watch the subject, you don't want it to get to be charisma and manipulation and not realise that they are having their strings pulled like public...so I hate that."

Seven clinicians expressed self-belief in their leadership capabilities and a confidence that 'their approach to leading was legitimate'. A further seven were able to express their drive and persistence in taking their ideas forward within their organisations and in one interview this drive and persistence had led to national dissemination of the individual's project. Humility emerged in two interviews in the form of those clinicians stepping-back and allowing others to receive recognition for their ideas. These two clinicians had gained satisfaction from the knowledge that their ideas and vision had been taken on by others, implemented and change had occurred.

Within the second theme, 'empowering others' emerged as an element of leadership development in eight interviews. As one clinician said:

> "I think that probably over the years I have tried to share the ideas with other people and somebody said that if you can really implement your ideas but at the same time make it feel as if it was theirs …that is where your thinking is going to succeed."

Seven clinicians expressed development of their ability to recognise the strengths and weaknesses of others and to build on the skills and competencies of others. These seven clinicians also had the elements of 'empowering others' and two described actively leading through people to deliver change. Awareness and attempts to adopt different leadership approaches emerged in nine interviews either by a broadened approach or adoption of different styles of leadership including a flexible style to accommodate different circumstances.

> "It does at times give you the ability to go for a bit about à la carte choice. You know you can choose your setting, your style, your manner, so you can change the things you do, although as a human being you flip back into your comfort zone whenever you can."

Working collaboratively with staff, stakeholders or other organisations emerged as an element in half of the interviews. Influencing at high levels within their organisation or the NHS emerged from three interviews. One clinician described his leadership style to be one of influencing at senior level within the organisation:

> "My preferred style is backstairs and to influence people. I'm good one-to-one. I'm very persuasive one-to-one and I can usually get my way one-to-one. I have to plan much harder if I'm going into an open forum and I usually do it by one-to-one conversations before you go into the forum."

> "I think I'm really quite influential…I have to have key relationships…I see myself as the planter to the power behind the throne…"

Political awareness emerged in two interviews where clinicians expressed a development in their ability to 'work with politics' and 'play the game'.

Critical incident stories

Critical incident reports are a method of seeking out details of specific events that have taken place as opposed to gathering people's generalisations, theories or impressions.

In Table 5.1, the themes emerging from each story are summarised. Fifteen out of the twenty examples were considered successful by the clinicians, including one pilot project. Three projects are on-going, two more did not give a clear indication of their success (Consultant Appraisal-clinician G, and Clinical Alliance-clinician J). One clinician (F) described strong personal gains from the MA throughout the interview and gave these as one of the examples. Two clinicians provided

Table 5.1: Summarised themes from critical incident reports

ID	First example	Second example
A	Directorate restructure Visionary, project leader, influencing, empowering, key stakeholder involvement, consulted widely, implemented and reviewed, cost effective. Successful	Solving a departmental problem Creative, project leader, facilitated, key stakeholders involved, empowered staff. Successful
B	Joint Mental Health Strategy Visionary, strategic, political awareness, broad approach, collaborative working, key stakeholder involvement, obtained external funding, Dissemination nationally. Successful	City wide strategy for a population subgroup with mental health problems Visionary, strategic, key stakeholder involvement, collaborative working, dissemination and implemented, obtained external funding, Successful
C	Introducing new departmental technology Innovative, visionary, project leader, strategic influencing, key stakeholder involvement, evidence-based approach, awaiting Trust ratification. Ongoing	Role extension of professionals allied to medicine Visionary, leading, empowered staff, influencing staff, modernising the department, skill mixing, implemented, reviewed, accountable for the staff and project. Successful
D	Modernised service delivery (Ward rounds) Visionary, innovative, project leader, key stakeholder involvement, empowering, driver for change, patient advocacy, influencing, implemented, reviewed, successful	Departmental modernisation Visionary, innovative, project leader, key stakeholder involvement, empowered staff, evidence-based approach, implemented, reviewed, obtained internal funding. Successful

(continued)

Table 5.1: Summarised themes from critical incident reports *(continued)*

ID	First example	Second example
E	Modernised service delivery for a population subgroup with mental health problems Visionary, strategic influencing, key stakeholder involvement, collaborative working, obtained external funding. Successful	Modernised service delivery (Ward based) Visionary, creative, leader within consultant body, strategic influencing, driver for change, implemented, accountability. Successful
F	Departmental transfer to PCT Strategic influencing, tactical, political awareness, personal integrity. Successfully maintained the team during transfer to new organisation	Personal survival during PCT transfer Self awareness, self belief, self development persistent, tactical skills, people management, awareness of others, valuing others, different leadership style
G	Introduced consultant appraisal Culture change within organisation, making staff feel valued, empowering, enabling and facilitating	Introduced clinical governance to merged directorate Led the process, creative, tactical methods, team building, empowering, developing a learning culture, influencing staff. Ongoing.
H	Risk management (out of hours cover) Identified the problem, creative, strategic influencing, political awareness, tactical methods, implemented with review. Successful	Driving change (consultant contract) Strategic vision, strategic influencing, strategic planning, networking, implementation Ongoing project but supported by Trust.
I	Health improvement (vaccination programme) Visionary, innovative, led the project, strategic influencing, key stakeholder involvement, driving change through people, empowering staff, communication the vision, submitted report, Successful	Health improvement programme (drinking water) Identified the problem, visionary, creative, strategic influencing, evidence based, piloted, key stakeholder involvement, tactical, involved the media, external funding, persistent. Successful pilot and ongoing project.
J	Modernised service delivery (clinical alliance) Medical lead, collaborative working, networking, spokesperson for Trust, implementation.	Improving working lives (mentoring system for doctors in training) Identified the need, visionary, creative, scanning, networking, communicated the vision, empowering staff. Successfully implemented.

validity to their examples by spontaneously providing written evidence to support their description. The examples demonstrated a range of benefits to the NHS, either nationally or locally, within individual Trusts or within departments.

Difficulties undertaking the MA

Difficulties experienced by clinicians undertaking the MA or criticisms of the course were not directly inquired about, but emerged during seven interviews. Criticisms were categorised into five categories and emerged in six interviews. One clinician did not rate the course leadership group and had difficulty relating to one tutor. A further clinician reported that other students did not rate the particular style of one of the tutors. Three clinicians indicated that the teaching did not cover particular skills and that the teaching did not equate to competency. Two clinicians considered ongoing coaching or mentoring, after the course ended, would have been useful. One clinician remained unconvinced about the evidence base.

Difficulties were categorised into four categories and emerged in six interviews. Three clinicians reported significant tensions between work commitments and course commitments, one of whose attendance on the course was significantly impaired. Two clinicians found difficulty committing time to the course. One clinician felt that self-motivation and self-direction were essential requirements for the course. Two clinicians described a negative effect on their personal and social life. Three clinicians were neither critical nor disclosed difficulties with the course.

Discussion

The concepts of management and leadership have been seen as almost interchangeable until the end of the twentieth century when authors converged on the notion that *management* was seen to be creating organisation, order and stability and *leadership* as creating energy, thrust, alignment, focus and commitment (Kent *et al.*, 2001). Kent *et al.* differentiate leading from managing in terms of why the two processes exist; what they produce or create, and how they are executed or carried out.

He describes *management* as allocating and insuring the effective use of resources in the accomplishment of organisational goals and *leadership* as marshalling, energising and unifying people towards the pursuit of a vision. Bennis (1998) differentiates between the leader and the manager by arguing that the leader masters the context as opposed to the manager who surrenders to it.

Both management and leadership are essential components to effective performance, modernisation, leading and implementing change, in any organisation. Egan (1993) argues that companies and institutions need to develop the systems to ensure a steady supply of good managers and leaders, with leaders developed throughout the organisation.

The new NHS Leadership Centre was created to deliver the promised 'step change in the calibre of NHS leadership'. The expectation is that managers will lead the modernisation programme and will require the development of managerial skills and leadership qualities – but also that there will be leaders at all levels in the NHS from those at the front-line to those in the most senior positions.

Leadership studies began to emerge from the 1930s and can be usefully described in four phases. These signal a change in emphasis rather than a demise of the previous approaches (Bryman, cited in McAreavey *et al.*, 2001):

1. The *Trait* approach (up to the late 1930s): Leaders are born rather than made, nature is more important than nurture;
2. The *Style* approach (late 1940s to the late 1960s): Behaviour of leaders is important;
3. The *Contingency* approach (late 1960s to early 1980s): Leaders can develop their skills and deploy them as the situation demands;
4. The *New leadership* approach (early 1980s onwards): the hybrid theories.

The *new leadership* approach encompassed a major paradigm shift from *transactional* models of leadership to *transformational* models. Burns (1978) described *transactional* leadership as the less desirable form involving motivation of followers by manipulative exchange using a reward system and *transformational* leadership as the engagement between leaders and followers leading to achievement of higher motivation and morality in both leaders and followers.

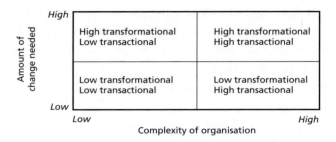

Figure 5.2: When different types of leadership are needed (Kotter, 1990

In practice, it is well recognised that there is no all-purpose leadership style. Instead successful leaders adapt their behaviour to meet the demands of different situations and different individuals (Connor, 2002). Edmonstone and Western (2002) argue that both transformational and transactional leaders are required within the NHS due to the high level of complexity of the organisation and the high amount of change required, based on Kotter's model illustrated in Figure 5.2.

Within the new leadership approach a further concept emerged, that of *servant leadership*, inspired by Greenleaf (cited in Russell, 2001) and suggesting that "leadership must first and foremost meet the needs of others".

Studies of leadership have also included the skills and qualities that effective leaders require. The more recent work by Alimo-Metcalfe and Alban-Metcalfe (2001, 2002) within the NHS and local government led to the development of the Transformational Leadership Questionnaire (TLQ) in an attempt to measure leadership within the UK public sector. The main components are listed in Box 5.2. The model 'significantly reflects aspects of the modernisation agenda' with an emphasis towards 'servant leadership' and is 'fundamentally about engaging others as partners in developing and achieving the shared vision, creating a supportive environment for creative thinking and challenging assumptions for healthcare delivery'.

The NHS Leadership Centre has developed the NHS Leadership Competencies Framework (2002) to describe the range of qualities required for leadership roles across the NHS. There are 15 qualities

Box 5.2: Components of TLQ

- Genuine concern for others
- Shows political sensitivity and skills
- Decisive displays, determined, self confident
- Empowers, develops potential
- Inspirational networker and promoter
- Accessible, approachable
- Clarifies boundaries, involves others in decisions
- Encourages critical and strategic thinking

grouped in 3 clusters (Figure 5.3). The *personal qualities* are at the core of the framework. *Setting the direction* refers to those qualities that enable the leader to set a vision for the future drawing on the understanding of the organisation in which they work, based on their political awareness of the health and social context. This is underpinned by their ability to move between the big picture vision and local operational detail, coupled

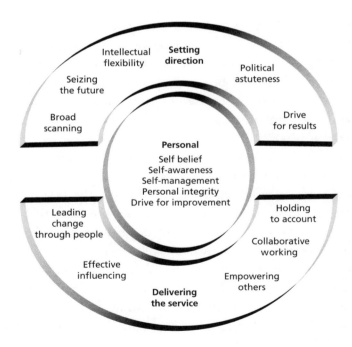

Figure 5.3: Leadership qualities framework

with their drive, inspiration and motivation of others. *Delivering the service* refers to range of styles and ways of working emphasising empowerment and partnership.

Experts on leadership and management development as far back as 1991 (Lyall, 1991) have called upon the NHS to "grow its own leaders" and warned that "it was essential for doctors to become involved in management" echoing the 1984 Griffiths Report.

When NHS Trusts were formed in 1991, doctors became more heavily involved in management. The statutory position of Medical Director (MD) was created and the role of the Clinical Director (CD) was introduced. MD duties have been clearly defined (BAMM, 2001) but the roles and responsibilities of CDs, who are non-statutory and who may control large budgets with a responsibility to manage medical colleagues, have only recently been highlighted (BAMM 2003). The selection of a CD has often been ad hoc, with no assessment of managerial competency, given token importance and, therefore, devalued – yet the role has expanded and taken on significant responsibilities (Bullock, 2002).

Training in management is a relatively recent phenomenon for doctors and was only introduced as mandatory for doctors in training in 1993. It is just beginning to emerge in undergraduate training (Davidson and Boggis, 2002). Clinicians taking on formal leadership/management roles such as MD or CD, tend to be more senior doctors who predate Calman training, who may have had no exposure to management training and who may be relatively poorly prepared for these roles (Bullock, 2002; McIntyre *et al.*, 2002).

With the emphasis now switched to a focus on leadership, leadership development programmes in the NHS are still in their infancy. Although there is a more co-ordinated approach through the NHS Leadership Centre, there remains little in the literature on the evaluation of leadership and management programmes for doctors. Historically, the NHS has focussed primarily on individual skill development with managers learning about leadership ideas and skills, delivered by externally-provided programmes and offering little which was specific to the local challenges facing individuals (Edmonstone and Western, 2002). Goodwin (cited in Edmonstone and Western, 2002) suggested that leadership development should be:

- Mandatory
- Locally-focused
- Based around Action Learning approaches
- Concentrated on inter-organisational and shared leadership between organisations, rather than 'leader/follower' relationships within organisations.

Edmonstone and Western (2002) identified a number of leadership development programmes (not specific to clinicians) ranging from national, regional, local and employer programmes to individual initiative programmes (MBA, postgraduate diplomas) with a range of funding from centrally funded to self-funded but with no cohesion or 'dovetailing' of the activity. The authors call for a more careful and judicious use of work-based and programme-based approaches that are subject to evaluation.

In this study, training in management/leadership emerged as one of the commonest reasons for applying for the MA, with half of the clinicians wanting training for a formal management or leadership role. The emphasis was towards training in management or change implementation as opposed to leadership training. Interestingly, training in elements of leadership was perceived as more beneficial for job effectiveness. One possible explanation for this could be due to confusion between management and leadership concepts prior to the course and the lack of clarity and definition surrounding the formal roles available to clinicians (in terms of management or leadership expectations). The course aims to provide a systematic approach to management and leadership, but the emphasis is on leadership development of the individual – and not on training in management. It should therefore, seem appropriate that leadership training was emphasised in the interviews.

The emphasis towards leadership also emerged within clinicians' roles, with the majority of clinicians' perceiving themselves as leaders and perceiving that their colleagues and team perceived them as leaders. The emphasis was towards leadership even when the perception was of both manager and leader:

> "I do one session management and within that management my role really is mostly a leadership role and a limited operational role."

Where the formal role contained management responsibilities these were frequently delegated to general managers who were not clinicians. Whether this is cause or effect from the MA, the preference to leadership over management was marked. Thorne (1997) argues this emphasis towards leadership and suggests that the formal role of Clinical Director should be expressed as leadership not management. Thorne also argues that managers exercise authority over subordinates but that leaders rely more heavily on influencing others to want to follow them and suggests that Clinical Directors are primarily change agents and shapers of meaning who influence others to follow a vision or a desired course of action. The themes emerging from my research would tend to support this argument. There is an emphasis towards leadership within roles, within the clinicians' development and within their projects. Influencing others is highlighted in the 'critical incident reports' and is considered as the only real power the clinicians' have in their formal roles. The term *manager* applied to the medical profession is indeed confusing. This research highlights the need to rethink the terminology and clarify and define formal roles for clinicians.

Several authors have emphasised the need for appropriate and relevant training in leadership and management for doctors (McIntyre *et al.*, 2002, Walker and Morgan, 1996, Edmonstone and Western, 2002). Although my sample size was small, there is confirmation that clinicians are still seeking appropriate training for formal roles in management/leadership and are taking on these roles without formal training. All of the clinicians in this study predated Calman training.

Emerging from the study are the perceptions that those who take on the formal roles consider that they may have some natural aptitude for the role but frequently that they may be the only clinician stepping forward. The general unpopularity of these roles can be identified from the emerging themes on the difficulties these clinicians have encountered in their formal or informal roles and with three clinicians moving away from the formal roles. This would confirm the work of other authors (Willcocks, 1997, Smith, 2001; McIntyre *et al.*, 2002; Bullock, 2002) who have cited similar difficulties with these roles such as insufficient time allocated to the role; conflict between management and clinical work; credibility both with peers and managers, insufficient support; power only by influence; and difficulties in engaging clinicians to change.

Bullock (2002) attempts to define the roles and characteristics of a good Clinical Director and provides a strong argument for acknowledgement, support and true recognition of the role, with the emphasis on "creating a true leadership role, not just a managerial one". BAMM (2003) has recently attempted to define the Clinical Director role. This research would further support the argument for rethinking the terminology and clarifying and defining formal roles for clinicians.

Over half the clinicians regarded the MA as having influenced their career progression in terms of role or job changes. My own perception of the data is that greater self-awareness and knowledge gained from the course had empowered the clinicians to make better-informed choices about their career progression.

The findings from this research have revealed that all the clinicians perceived that they had developed as leaders and that elements of transformational, situational and servant leadership were present within this development. In addition, a range of qualities emerged from the 'critical incident reports' with clinicians displaying innovative and creative ideas; using their influence to communicate and engage staff and senior management; empowering staff; collaborating and working in partnerships and implementing their ideas with review and evaluation. These correlate with the desirable elements of transformational leaders from the work of Alimo-Metcalfe and Alban-Metcalfe (2001, 2002).

In comparison, between the findings from this study and the Leadership Qualities Framework (LQF), self-awareness, personal integrity and self-belief emerged as personal qualities from a high proportion of the interviews. A significant number of the clinicians were able to express their drive and persistence in taking their ideas forward within their organisations. Political astuteness was apparent within the 'critical incident reports' with the focus more on 'in-house politics' and playing the political game of their own organisations. Collaborative working, empowering and influencing others emerged strongly from the 'reports'. A number also developed their projects through other people – 'leading change through people'. In addition, a broadened leadership approach, flexible styles, elements of transactional, transformational and servant leadership emerged in the interviews.

The findings from this research would suggest that the MALIC has been perceived to develop the clinicians as leaders and that their "individual potential" has been enhanced.

All ten doctors perceived the MA to have had a positive influence on themselves or their ability to perform their roles more effectively. Training has already been highlighted. The use of the theory from the course was highlighted as being of practical benefit and 'always in the background'. Theory is essential grounding knowledge for a subject, providing the basic understanding and always present as an anchor and reference. The ability of the clinicians to apply the theory into practice is captured within the 'reports' and can provide some evidence of their effectiveness. The skills acquired from the course included being able to manage people and confidence. These are likely to be beneficial to their effectiveness as managers/leaders. Leaders need to be self-aware and have an awareness of others. Self-reflection is therefore crucial to developing individuals, as is recognising strengths and weaknesses. The majority of clinicians acknowledged this as important. The opportunity to network enabled the clinicians to have contacts, role models and coaching. Specific issues relating to their own work could be brought to course groups discussed, brain-stormed and problem-solved. These could then be applied back to their own organisations with obvious benefits.

The intention of this study was not to evaluate the course programme and the findings of my research cannot be used to evaluate the programme. However, the perceived benefits of academic study included protected study time, time out from work, in-depth study and acquiring new research skills. Only three clinicians highlighted the actual qualification as desirable. I believe this suggests that it is the course programme that is attractive, as opposed to another qualification for clinicians who are already highly-trained and qualified. The negative sides of the programme are the time-commitment; the requirement to balance clinical, managerial and study commitments; and the effect that this has on personal and social lives.

The programme involves a small group of individuals (clinicians, managers, leaders) chosen through interview in an attempt to balance skills and backgrounds, break down barriers and to foster a learning culture based around Action Learning. The learning and teaching styles are not suited to everyone and should be a consideration at interview. The closeness of the groups can also create difficulties if personalities and styles are not suited. The programme is leadership-focused and follows the philosophy of the NHS Leadership Centre in suggesting that participants should develop the skills required to lead the modernisation programme.

Conclusions

In drawing my conclusions from this research, my feeling is that there was a significant perceived impact of the MALIC in all the three areas explored. Leadership appears more strongly emphasised as the role the clinicians have adopted either informally or formally. All the clinicians perceived that they had developed as leaders with greater self-awareness and confidence in their skills. This would suggest that "individual potential" has been enhanced following the MA – one of the stated aims of the course.

The data are rich with the perceived positive benefits for the individual clinicians in their roles at work, the skills they have acquired to perform their roles and their personal development. Acquiring knowledge of the relevant theory and the application of this to practice, coupled with the skill and personal development is likely to be beneficial to the organisations these individuals work in. All the clinicians gave examples of personal leadership in areas of innovation and change within their organisations, suggesting opportunities for organisational enhancement, a further stated aim of the course.

This research highlights the need to rethink the terminology and clarify and define formal management and leadership roles for clinicians. The research also highlights the continuing difficulties of clinicians undertaking formal roles that are not supported or truly valued and without appropriate training.

My perception from this study is that the themes emerging suggest that the MALIC course can develop the qualities required for clinician leaders within the NHS who should be able to deliver the modernisation agenda.

This study has explored the perceptions of clinicians after the course and would have been greatly enhanced by an assessment of their skills and competencies prior to the course. The study would also have benefited from independent correlation of the emergent themes through exploring the perceptions of the staff, peers and senior management within the organisations.

Recommendations derived from this study include that:

- Future evaluation of leadership training and development programmes for clinicians can be enhanced by assessing skills and competencies of potential candidates prior to the programme and after completion. Evaluations should also incorporate the views of staff, peers or senior managers from within the potential candidates' organisation.
- Interviews for the MALIC course could incorporate the suitability of the teaching and learning styles for potential candidates.
- Methods for facilitating ongoing coaching and mentoring following the MALIC course should be considered. This could also apply to other leadership programmes.
- Formal roles of management and leadership for clinicians should be clearly-defined and renamed to reflect the emphasis on leadership.
- Formal roles for clinicians should be acknowledged, supported, and valued within organisations.
- Clinicians predating Calman Training who wish to consider formal roles should be offered appropriate training, support and opportunities for self-reflection.
- Clinicians considering formal roles should be assessed for their suitability within a formal process.
- Succession planning for formal roles for clinicians needs to be addressed with some urgency within the NHS.

References

Alimo-Metcalfe, B. & Lawler, J. (2001) "Leadership development in UK companies at the beginning of the twenty-first century", *Journal of Management in Medicine,* Vol. 15, No. 5, pp 387–404.

Alimo-Metcalfe, B. & Alban-Metcalfe, J. (2002) "Leadership: half the battle", *Health Service Journal,* Vol. 112, No. 5795, pp 26–27.

Bennis, W. (1998) *On Becoming a Leader,* London, Arrow Books.

British Association of Medical Managers (2001) *The Duties of the Medical Director,* Stockport, British Association of Medical Managers.

British Association of Medical Managers (2003) *The Roles and Responsibilities of the Clinical Director,* Stockport, British Association of Medical Managers.

Bullock, R. (2002) "Can Damocles rediscover Hippocrates?: what is the developing role of the clinical director?", *Clinician in Management*, Vol. 11, No. 2, pp 61–66.

Burns, J. (1978) *Leadership*, New York, Harper & Row.

Connor, M. (2002) "Situational leadership in practice", *MA in Leadership, Innovation and Change*.

Davidson, C. & Boggis, C. (2002) "Management for medical students", *Clinician in Management*, Vol. 11, No. 4, pp 177–80.

Davies, H. & Harrison, S. (2003) "Trends in doctor–manager relationships" *British Medical Journal*, Vol. 326, No. 7390, pp 646–649.

Degeling, P., Maxwell, S., Kennedy, J. & Coyle, B. (2002) "Medicine, management and modernisation: a 'danse macabre'?" *British Medical Journal* Vol. 326, No. 7390, pp 649–652.

Denscombe, M. (1998) *The Good Research Guide,* Buckingham, Open University Press.

Department of Health (1993) *Hospital Doctors: Training for the Future,* London, The Stationery Office.

Department of Health (2001) *Shifting the Balance of Power within the NHS: Securing Delivery,* London, The Stationery Office.

Department of Health (2000) *The NHS Plan: A Plan for Investment: A Plan for Reform,* London, The Stationery Office.

Department of Health (2002) *Delivering the NHS Plan: Next Steps on Investment: Next Steps on Reform,* London, The Stationery Office.

Edmonstone, J. & Western, J. (2002) "Leadership development in healthcare: what do we know?", *Journal of Management in Medicine*, Vol. 16, No. 1, pp 34–47.

Egan, G. (1993) *Adding Value,* San Francisco, Jossey-Bass.

Gaughan, A. (2001) "Effective leadership behaviour: leading the 'third way' from a Primary Care Group perspective: a study of leadership constructs elicited from members of Primary Care Group management boards", *Journal of Management in Medicine*, Vol. 15, No. 1, pp 67–94.

Kent, T., Crotts, J. & Azziz, A. (2001) "Four factors of transformational leadership behaviour", *Leadership and Organisation Development Journal,* Vol. 22, No. 5, pp 221–229.

Lyall, J. (1991) "Top managers: the NHS must grow its own", *Health Manpower Management*, Vol. 17, No. 2, pp 4–5.

McAreavey, M., Alimo-Metcalfe, B. & Connelly, J. (2001) "How do directors of public health perceive leadership?", *Journal of Management in Medicine*, Vol. 15, No. 6, pp 446–462.

McIntyre, H., Graham, B. & Wray, R. (2002) "Is the role of clinical director bound to fail?" *Clinician in Management*, Vol. 11, No. 4, pp 163–167.

Mason, M. (1996) *Qualitative Researching*, London, Sage.

NHS Leadership Centre (2002) *NHS Leadership Qualities Framework*, NHS Modernisation Agency.

Russell, R.F. (2001) "The role of values in servant leadership", *Leadership & Organisation Development Journal*, Vol. 22, No. 2, pp 76–83.

Smith, D. (2001) 'Why are doctors unhappy?" *British Medical Journal* , Vol. 322, pp 1073–1074.

Thorne, M. (1997) 'Myth management in the NHS", *Journal of Management in Medicine*, Vol. 11, No. 3, pp 168–180.

Walker, R. & Morgan, P. (1996) "Involving doctors in management", *Journal of Management in Medicine*, Vol. 10, No. 1, pp 31–52.

Wengraf, T. (2001) *Qualitative Research Interviewing*, London, Sage.

Willcocks, S. (1997) "Managerial effectiveness in the NHS. A possible framework for considering the effectiveness of the clinical director", *Journal of Management in Medicine*, Vol. 11, No. 3, pp 181–189.

CHAPTER SIX

GP leadership development in the Northern Deanery

Julia Pokora, Alan Phillips & Tim van Zwanenberg

Three strategic themes have been proposed for the future development of general medical practice, namely:

1. *Leadership* to embrace and lead change,
2. *Scholarship* for intellectual stimulation, and
3. *Fellowship* for mutual support. (van Zwanenberg, 1998)

In a system such as general practice, predicated on peer relationships, the notion of leadership may appear counter-intuitive. Leadership, however, is a function much needed by organisations at times of turbulence, for leaders can empower and enable others to harness and implement change. The former Chief Medical Officer for England said that " leadership requires knowing where you want to go, taking people with you, and giving sufficient time and energy to make it happen" (Calman, 1998).

This latter aspect of leadership, that of promoting organisational development, is much needed in primary care at the moment (Koeck, 1998).The Government has recognised that its reform of the NHS will require first class leaders at all levels, though priority for action on leadership development has gone in the first instance to hospitals rather than primary care. (DoH, 2000). In fact the notion of a "primary care-led" NHS was first mooted in the mid-1990s, yet arguably little has been done to develop leadership appropriately among general practitioners and other primary care personnel. The idea of leadership development for general practitioners is not new. About 20 years ago quite large numbers of general practitioners went on the "MSD programme" devised by

Professor Marshall Marinker, and sponsored by the pharmaceutical company Merck, Sharpe and Dome. That course was originally designed to develop participants' small group leadership skills. The programme organisers, however, quickly realised that the participants were developing more generic leadership skills (personal communication – M Marinker).

It is some years since those courses were run, and yet the pace of change in primary care has accelerated not diminished. Now general practitioners are developing new roles as "GP specialists" and in the corporate management of primary care, as well as adjusting their traditional roles in providing acute consumer-responsive care and continuing relationship-based care (van Zwanenberg, 2001). The development of leadership among general practitioners remains a most pressing requirement.

This chapter describes our approach and experience from running a modular residential leadership development programme for the "new generation of GP leaders" in the Northern Deanery over the last three years. Armed with the lessons from this programme we are now embarking on a programme of inter-professional leadership development in primary care.

The programme design

Unhappily, many leadership development initiatives, in common with most change programmes, fail to deliver the desired outcomes (Egan, 1993).

The increasing emphasis in the NHS and elsewhere on "outside–in" leadership development may be a significant factor in this failure. Whilst intended to facilitate leadership development, it appears to have the reverse effect. Outside- in leadership development starts with, and subsequently emphasises, the requirements of the leadership role. A set of qualities or characteristics, the profile of the "ideal" leader is produced. Participants are invited to measure themselves against this profile, and address performance deficits. Thus, leadership development is seen as training to acquire a set of skills and abilities. Over recent years, the competency framework, one version of this approach, has proved appealing and popular. Whilst its limitations have been noted (Burgoyne, 1990), the approach is seductive in its apparent scientific rationality. It continues to influence leadership development, even though the evidence base for the competencies may be unclear. Moreover, the approach is theory-centred not learner-centred. It can increase pressure on already anxious participants, concerned about whether they "measure up" to the leadership profile. Such a reaction is not conducive to learning and development.

Another version of "outside-in" occurs when leadership is described as something larger-than-life, a heroic activity and the province of great men and women, often political or military figures. Whilst intended to inspire, the impact of this approach can be the reverse, setting apart leadership in the minds of participants as something "other than" and different from themselves.

A third variation comes in the form of over-reliance on one leadership model or framework. Tichy and Ulrich used the phrase "transformational leader" to describe a dynamic, visionary style of leadership in contrast to more conventional ("transactional") leadership – see Table 6.1 (Tichy & Ulrich, 1984). This useful elaboration has influenced leadership development in a less useful way. The (more fashionable) attributes of transformational leadership are given pre-eminence, and transformational and transactional behaviours are described as two different personality types, so that participants are exhorted to become more like a "transformational" leader. Recent research (Alimo-Metcalfe & Alban-Metcalfe, 2000) has questioned the applicability of this model to the UK and to the NHS. However it remains influential.

Whilst the outside-in perspective is important, over-emphasising it can result in leadership development losing sight of some essential truths

Table 6.1: Transformational v transactional leadership

Transactional leadership	Transformational leadership
• Head down	• Head up
• Focus on practical	• Focus on possible
• Doing the job right	• Doing the right job
• Sets objectives	• Questions assumptions
• Fixes problems	• Creates problems
• Directs energy	• Creates energy
• Turns ideas into reality	• Stimulates ideas
• Coaches performance	• Inspires potential
• Pragmatic	• Visionary

about human nature and about how adults learn. We consider that self-understanding in the essential pre-requisite to and first step in leadership development. Moreover, leadership education must move beyond competency towards *capability* – "the ability to adapt to change, generate new knowledge and continuously improve performance" (Fraser & Greenhalgh, 2000).

Against this background the development programme for general practitioners was guided by the following assumptions:

1. Leadership development is something more than the acquisition of a set of skills and competencies. It is a process involving the whole person and their exploration of beliefs, attitudes, values, capabilities and preferences (Bennis & Nanus, 1997).

2. Leadership development is a journey, a path to becoming the best leader you can be. One function of a leadership development programme is to provide a "map" and way-markers for participants to locate themselves in their journey, to see where they have come from, to understand the terrain and to plan their future direction.

3. Leadership development involves both the "inner" and the "outer". The "inner" includes all the things which define the person, and which they take into their work including their skills, experience, values, beliefs, and aims. "Outer" includes all the external influences, which shape a person's leadership, including the demands of the role, the key stakeholders, the local and national agenda and future trends (see Figure 6.1).

4. Leadership development requires a balance of support and challenge. Participants must feel they are working in a safe confidential environment where they will be respected. They need to understand and value the things they do well. To develop, they also need challenge from new ideas, different perspectives and feedback from others.

5. Leadership development requires a balance of reflection and action. Structured (and unstructured) reflection on experiences within and outside the programme is encouraged, so that participants can discover

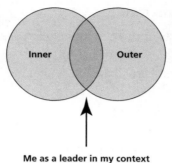

All the things that define the person I am and which I bring to work each day:

- history, skills and experiences
- values and feelings
- personality
- personal goals and vision
- life outside work

All the influences from the world around me that shape how I work as a professional and leader:

- demands and challenges
- stakeholders ... people I work for and with
- change agenda
- local influences
- national and political context

Me as a leader in my context

Figure 6.1: Leadership development – working with the inner and the outer

the themes and patterns of their leadership. This is a key part of the development process, because it enables participants to challenge themselves, which creates a powerful force for change – often more powerful than challenge from others. The programme, in addition, requires participants to try out ideas back at work and report the outcomes.

6. Leadership development is a social as well as a personal process. The programme aims to build a learning network and learning relationships whose life extends beyond the boundaries of the programme. It addresses all four levels of learning (see Table 6.2). Participants acquire knowledge about leadership, about the NHS and about themselves. They develop new skills and behaviours, which reflect new attitudes and perceptions. They consider what they want to become, and how best to fulfil their potential. They learn together, and consider their impact on the Deanery and local organisations. It is at this level of collaborative enquiry that inroads into organisational learning are made.

Table 6.2: Levels of Learning (after Pedler and Aspinwall, 1996)

1. Knowledge.....about things
2. Skills and abilities....to do
3. Potential...personal development
4. Acting together....collaborative enquiry

The programme structure

The programme consists of three modules, each separated by four weeks, so that it runs over a three-month period. Each programme has a maximum of 12 participants. Participants have included:

- Chairs of Primary Care Groups
- Clinical Leads
- General practitioners who, whilst not in a formal leadership role, are involved in local service developments
- General practitioners who wish to play a more prominent and effective role in the leadership of their practice.

The first module focuses primarily upon intensive *personal diagnosis*. The overall framework of the programme is described, and ideas about leadership and the NHS context introduced. Participants undertake a review of themselves and their values, beliefs, strengths and development needs in relationship to leadership. They formulate a personal definition of leadership, and begin the process of planning their development.

The second module focuses upon *acting strategically as a leader* in primary care. Topics include thinking and acting purposefully to achieve strategic impact, and skilful influencing.

The third module focuses on *leading and managing organisation change*. Participants consider both their personal and their organisational development goals, and their plans to achieve these.

This programme is flexible, and there is ongoing review and formative feedback at each stage, so that it can be tailored to respond to participants' needs. Participants are encouraged to take responsibility for their own learning, and various development assignments during the modules and between modules encourage them to do this.

A variety of learning methods are used. In addition to plenary, small group and pairs work, each participant has at least two one-to-one development sessions with a facilitator. Work is sometimes structured around participants' work issues, sometimes around a theory or framework, and in addition external speakers contribute to sessions. Other learning methods include a psychometric inventory, learning journals, mentoring and the development of learning partnerships.

Programme evaluation

Postal questionnaires were sent to participants from the first three programmes, and 76.5% (26 out of 34) were returned. The questionnaire contained seven open questions about the impact of the programme. By using this open-ended approach, we intended to maximise the amount of qualitative information received.

The questions focused on:

A. Whether participants had become aware of changes in the way they exercised or thought about leadership
B. The impact (if any) the programme had produced on their working lives
C. The impact (if any) on them more personally
D. The most important aspects of the learning process and content.

The responses, which were rich in detail and narrative, were analysed, and a number of clear themes emerged. These are summarised below.

Changes in leadership thinking/behaviour

Several themes emerged in relation to how participants *thought about* and *exercised* leadership.

There was an appreciation that a wide range of leadership styles might be effective but particularly the possibility that a facilitative style might be productive, in contrast to the traditional "command and control" approach. Participants noted that skills of active listening, of influencing and persuading, of encouraging and supporting, were proving important to them in bringing about change in their practices and beyond.

> "Much more confident that *my form* of leadership – facilitative, encouraging others – is valid and useful".

> "(I've put) more effort into trying to obtain opinions and ideas from ALL levels of the staff team. This has been worthwhile. Not 'compromise' but 'developing a better model'. I recognise that my quiet way of leading/encouraging development in others is effective leadership".

> "I am increasingly convinced that developing a healthy culture in an organisation will deliver much more than any other initiative. As a leader I think I have an important role to play in establishing a culture…"

One participant suggested that this style might be especially appropriate to primary care in its current stage of development.

> "In primary care organisations I think that 'leadership by service' is the only way to go. Anyone who attempts a dictatorial type of leadership will only put backs up…. I think a PCO really needs a lot of people putting in their piece of the jigsaw, and a 'leader' needs to facilitate this occurring."

Supporting this venture into facilitative leadership, there was for a number of participants a greater sense of self-confidence and self-awareness – confidence to be a leader, confidence to do it in their own way and awareness of their personal strengths and blind-spots, and their impact on others.

> "I'm not intimidated by the concept of leadership.."

> "I feel more relaxed about my role. Not feeling I have to have the answers but motivating, supporting and creating the environment for others. Insight into myself on this…Feel less pressured about my role within PCT, yet achieve as much as if dotting i's and crossing t's".

> "I think I feel more confident in leading in my own style rather than subconsciously emulating the style of others and finding it doesn't feel right. I'm now more conscious that my personality type influences my style of leadership.."

Lastly, there was a sense in which, for some participants, leadership had been brought within reach by the programme, not just the domain of the great man or woman but something that ordinary mortals could aspire to…echoing Egan's distinction between leadership and "headship" (Egan, 1993).

> "Leadership – not such a big word."

> "Leadership isn't rocket science."

Impact on working lives

All participants described a positive impact on their working lives. Some had become involved in the formal leadership of primary care (via Primary Care Groups/Trusts) and the processes of organisational change that accompany it:

> "Have reduced my clinical commitment in order to become Chair of PEC...It is clearly a leadership role.."

> "I've set up groups within the PCG to look at issues which have been causing conflict (e.g. resource allocation to practices).

> "I've co-authored the local IMT strategy, implemented a data quality project and set up IM&T structures for the PCT."

Others had worked within their practices to improve working methods and processes, and to improve working relationships:

> "...it has been a time of huge change within the Practice (instigating structural, personnel and IT change) and more broadly changing the ethos of the practice team, making everyone happier, more positive and forward-looking and an a more cohesive team with better communication."

> "Major impact. Frustration to calm; impasse to progress; stagnation to changes (multiple clinical and organisational)."

Others reported that, although not necessarily leading major change, they were working differently. They were more assertive, used a wider range of interpersonal skills to develop better working relationships with colleagues and used different approaches to solving problems.

> "The practice now has a much more confident, slightly more assertive GP who has skills ideally suited to her roles."

> "I'm more aware of other peoples' needs and how I can try and meet them. I've tried harder to show other people that I'm listening to them and valuing their view/contribution."

> "As a leader: I am less likely to 'flex my muscle' when influencing change. I spend more time considering when to direct and when to facilitate. I am more sensitive to the needs of ownership. Finally, I am more likely to weigh up other influences and then make decisions

about my further action. Previously I accepted some dictates without expression of my own judgement and on other occasions would jump to my own conclusions."

Personal impact

Participants reported increases in self-confidence, zest, enthusiasm and feelings of empowerment.

"The most lasting impact was: more confidence, self-belief and feeling that 'I'm okay.'"

"The most lasting impact was, I suppose, a feeling of empowerment."

"(It) boosted my enthusiasm for work again."

Some participants reported that the impact had spilled over the boundaries of their professional roles into their personal lives. They described being able to cope better with changes in life outside the work role and, in particular, of achieving a better balance between work and home life .

"Much more self-aware, settled and secure. Happier about work/life balance. Overall very positive."

"I have coped with tremendous changes in my personal life…. much better than I would have thought possible, and this is due to looking at problems more logically."

Learning process and content

Many participants reported on the characteristics of the learning process which had been significant in helping them to develop in the ways described above. First, it was an *"adult learning process"*, as one general practitioner put it, providing lots of flexibility, using a participative style, so that participants were fully involved in every way and able to influence the content and shape of the programme.

Second, much of the learning involved working closely with peers as "comrades in adversity" (Revans, 1998). Participants found it liberating to discover that colleagues had similar problems and similar difficulties in finding solutions. Peer support, encouragement and challenge were powerful in helping them to reframe and rethink problems and their impact on problems. This collaborative learning process served to counter the isolation often experienced by those working in primary care. It also modelled for participants a different, more interactive, way of working within the practice itself.

> "Buzzing people, buzzing ideas!"

> "..the protected time in an ideal environment with like-minded GPs to learn important skills and help us with our work/life balance."

> "..the opportunity to take time out to consider Practice problems with support and challenge, to look at ways forward and to see problems in perspective of others' Practices."

Third, participants valued working with both the "inner and the outer". Working with personal and organisational issues, and identifying connections between them proved to be a potent mixture and led, for some , to profound learning.

> "..it was excellent and coincided with a time in my life when change was being contemplated – this helped the strategy to evolve."

Finally, of the course content, participants particularly valued the Myers Briggs Type Indicator and the opportunity to look at themselves in some depth. This led to learning about how "the person I am" impacts upon different aspects of working life and particularly upon leadership style, preferences and potential blind spots. As one participant said:

> "Personal development is very important – and involves so much more than PGEA events and reading."

Discussion

It appears that self-awareness is at the core of leadership and leadership development. It has been said that *"Developing as a leader is much like developing as an integrated human being."* (Goleman, 1996). Good leaders understand themselves, they develop the ability to understand the behaviour of others and, crucially, to build effective working *relationships*. They have "emotional intelligence" The programme has strengthened this capability within the participants and they have both welcomed this and found it essential in effectively leading organisation change. There is support for the assumption that successful development starts by building confidence and building on strengths, rather than by identifying deficiencies, in participants. This strategy *energised* participants, who were then more inclined to take an active approach to their leadership development and, in time, to focus energy on dealing with their "blind-spots". It reduced the resistance often experienced by participants confronted with the "challenge of leadership", and/or performance deficiencies.

The significant investment in a three module residential programme over seven days has been important to provide participants with a "space" away from their daily work, in which they can engage in a process of personal reflection, rethinking themselves and their relation to the world they work in. It has proved an essential counterbalance to an NHS workplace that grows daily more intense, and a conclusion may be that productive *sustainable* change requires time and space.

Another source of learning has been the benefit of what one participant called an "adult learning process". The flexible programme has helped people to integrate new ideas with the reality of their working experience. It is a collaboration between facilitators and participants, building a learning community of peers. The process of leadership development is not something done *unto* participants, rather it is an offer to accompany them on a journey. Frequently, participants' previous experience of learning has been largely didactic and pedagogic, and they have found this very different process stimulating and energising.

If the NHS is really to be led from primary care, it would seem incongruous to develop leaders by imposing upon them a model of leadership formulated elsewhere. A more powerful option is to bring together potential leaders, in a spirit of collaborative enquiry, to develop an approach to leadership that both suits the primary care context and to which each person can contribute with self- belief and enthusiasm, in unique and individual ways.

Individuals choose to make leadership contributions in different ways. By valuing and supporting these contributions equally, an increasing number of general practitioners may be willing to see themselves as genuine leaders. In turn this means that leadership development will help to create a deep *capability* for leadership and change in the GP community, which will benefit primary care for many years to come. Leadership development is not only about developing the "stars" or those in formal leadership roles but rather about developing a broad leadership capability within the primary care system.

Perhaps, at the very least, we are producing a cohort of people who represent a *capability for change* within primary care. Some will lead change from formal positions of power and influence, whilst some will quietly introduce and facilitate changes in their practice and in local services. Others will simply cope with change better themselves and help others in their practices to do likewise, by virtue of their attitudes, their changed ways of thinking and working, and of relating to people.

References

Alimo-Metcalfe, B. & Alban-Metcalfe, R. (2000) "Heaven can wait", *Health Service Journal* (12th October).

Bennis, W. & Nanus, B. (1997) *Leaders – Strategies for Taking Charge (2nd Edition)* New York, HarperBusiness.

Burgoyne, J (1990) "Doubts about competency", Chapter 2 in Devine, M (ed.) *The Photofit Manager,* London, Unwin Hall.

Calman, K. (1998) "Lessons from Whitehall", *British Medical Journal,* No. 317, pp 1718–1720.

Department of Health (2000) *The NHS Plan: A Plan for Investment, a Plan for Reform*, London, The Stationery Office.

Egan, G. (1993) *Adding Value,* California, Jossey-Bass.

Fraser, S. & Greenhalgh, T. (2000) "Coping with complexity: educating for capability", *British Medical Journal,* No. 223: pp 799–803.

Goleman, D. (1996) *Emotional Intelligence*, London, Bloomsbury.

Koeck, C. (1998) "Time for organisational development in healthcare organisations", *British Medical Journal,* No. 317, pp 1267–1268.

Pedler, M. & Aspinwall, K (1996) *Perfect plc: The Purpose and Practice of Organisational Learning,* Maidenhead, McGraw-Hill.

Revans, R (1998) *The ABC of Action Learning*, London, Lemos & Crane.

Tichy, N. & Ulrich, D. (1984) "The leadership challenge: a call for transformational leadership", *Sloan Management Review,* Vol 26, No. 1.

van Zwanenberg, T. (2001) "The new GP", in Harrison, J, Innes, R & van Zwanenberg, T (eds.) *The New GP: Changing Roles and the Modern NHS,* Oxford, Radcliffe Medical Press.

van Zwanenberg, T. (1998) "GP tomorrow", in Harrison, J. & van Zwanenberg, T. (eds) *GP Tomorrow,* Oxford, Radcliffe Medical Press.

CHAPTER SEVEN

The Royal College of Nursing Clinical Leadership Programme

Geraldine Cunningham and Hazel Mackenzie

This chapter will cover the historical background, overview, design and impact of the Royal College of Nursing Clinical Leadership Programme. It will conclude by focussing on the Programme's future direction.

Introduction and historical background

A number of key issues faced nursing, nurses, patients and the wider health service in the early 1990s. In particular, patient satisfaction, relationships between ward leaders and quality of care, and an expansion of the demands on the ward leader role indicated the need for change and for fresh approaches to leadership development. At the time it was less clear, however, what the nature and focus of the new approach was to be.

It was against this background that in 1993, the Royal College of Nursing embarked on a programme of work that endeavoured to provide such clarity. The programme had a number of separate project strands underpinned by a belief that leadership skills are a requisite for all nurses who lead a team or group, from Staff Nurses to Directors of Nursing. Thus all nurses in positions requiring leadership skills should have the opportunity to develop their potential. One of the projects in this RCN portfolio arose directly from patient and carer expectations and directly linked to the leadership agenda. Key to the impetus for this discrete project was the assertion that patients and their families should be able to expect high standards of care, delivered by kind, understanding and professional nurses at the beside.

The RCN Ward Nursing Leadership Project (RCN, 1997, Cunningham & Kitson, 2000, Parts 1 and 2) was an action research project that ran from November, 1994 through to October, 1997 and was funded by a charitable trust. It was clear from existing research that the role of the Ward Sister/Charge Nurse was pivotal in determining the quality of care delivered within the ward. Good leaders produced good care and poor leaders produced poor care. The RCN Ward Nursing Leadership Project focused on the ward leader and their leadership qualities. The Project aimed to promote better practice by identifying the skills needed by ward leaders to make them more effective, then demonstrating how those skills could then be transferred to other nurses and make a positive impact on patient care. One of the strongest messages to emerge from the Project was that, although organisations can influence the quality of patient care, it is the qualities of individual nurses which have a more direct effect on the way that patients are looked after.

What started as an action research project involving four NHS Trusts in England, has now evolved into an international programme. Over 2,000 participants have now completed the RCN Clinical Leadership Programme which is running in over 160 healthcare organisations across England, Wales, Scotland, Belgium, Switzerland and Australia. Participants on the programme come from a variety of clinical backgrounds; including hospital nurses, community nurses, doctors, and allied health professionals.

The Programme has developed over three distinct phases since its inception. *Phase one* focused on exploring the leadership skills, techniques and talents required by clinical leaders to become more patients focused. A number of interventions were introduced and facilitated with the clinical leaders – 360° leadership feedback, personal development planning, mentorship, one-to-one supervision with the facilitator, needs led workshops, patient stories and observations of care. The data was qualitatively and quantitatively analysed. The results were positive, demonstrating a shift in leadership styles and organisation of care to be more patient-focused. From the qualitative data, five themes emerged to form the Clinical Leadership Framework that is now the foundation of the Programme.

- Learning to manage self
- Developing effective relationships
- Patient focus
- Networking
- Political awareness.   (RCN, 1997)

On completion of the first phase the Programme received an award in 1998, in recognition of being an outstanding health services management development innovation – the "Baxter Award for Excellence in Management Development".

One of the major challenges of the first phase of the research was the contention that the facilitator had made the difference and not the approach and interventions used, therefore deeming the Programme not replicable. This challenge led to the development of the second phase. At this point the name of the Programme changed to the RCN Clinical Leadership Programme as numerous clinical settings and disciplines became involved.

The *second phase* focused on translating the interventions used in the first phase into a tool-kit. The tool-kit was then used as the framework for the roll out of the Programme with 35 facilitators from NHS Trusts in England, Scotland and Wales. The aim was to evaluate the tool-kit and find out if the study could be replicated using different facilitators. The results did demonstrate that the Programme could be replicated with similar results to the first phase (Cunningham *et al.*, 2002).

The *third phase* involved 96 Programmes delivered in England funded by the National Nursing Leadership Project and included a multiple case study evaluation of the Programme, which enabled detailed analysis of the clinical leaders' journey through the Programme and the impact of that experience and the acceptability of the interventions. This was due to be completed in November 2003. The third phase also included nine Trusts in Scotland funded by the Scottish Executive and an evaluation study (MacKenzie and Cunningham, 2002).

Theoretical overview

The theoretical background of the RCN Ward Nursing Leadership Project was influenced strongly by humanistic theories of nursing practice, based on the work of a number of nurse theorists (Peplau 1952, Orem 1980, Henderson 1966), These influenced the initial design in the Project and the facilitation work of Kitson *et al.* (1996) and Heron (1989) and the seminal work of Menzies (1970) underpinned the facilitation of nurses' professional and personal development through collaboration with practitioners. In addition the humanistic theories appeared to link most closely to transformational leadership.

Burns (1978) first popularised the term of *transformational leadership* describing it as occurring when one or more persons engage with each other in such a way that leaders and followers raise one another to higher levels of motivation and morality. By utilising a variety of strategies including self-awareness, values and a vision for the future, leaders have a transforming effect on their followers, themselves and their organisations. Kouzes and Posner (1997) further this theme in their work by describing leadership as a performing art – a collection of practises and behaviours – rather than a position. They argue that excellence rises from within and cannot be imposed from without. They define leadership as

> "the art of mobilising others to want to struggle for shared aspirations"
>
> Kouzes & Posner, 1997

These theories have been supported by a more recent study (Alimo-Metcalfe & Alban-Metcalfe, 2000) undertaken on 2,000 NHS managers. This study suggested that the most important characteristics of effective leaders are concern for others and the ability to communicate and inspire. The picture that emerged was one that highlighted the complexity of the leadership roles in the NHS. Alimo-Metcalfe and Alban-Metcalfe conclude that while the transactional competencies of *management* are crucial they are simply not sufficient on their own. NHS organisations therefore must be willing to adapt and be truly committed to incorporating transformational leadership into their recruitment, selection, promotion, performance management and development processes for all staff, whatever their area or level of work.

Programme design

This section will focus on the Programme design and delivery, addressing aims, objectives and outcomes; establishing the programme; interventions and evaluation of the Programme.

The Programmes delivered by the RCN Clinical Leadership team incorporate the principles of transformational leadership (Bass, 1985; Bass & Avolio 1994) and lifelong learning (Revans, 1998). They are founded on research evidence and a value system that embraces the following beliefs:

- Effective leaders provide high quality patient/client care.
- All health and social care practitioners require leadership capabilities.
- It is possible for individuals to develop their leadership capabilities.
- Potential is best developed in a culture of high support and high challenge.
- Participants bring rich and varied experience to the Programmes. The strengths of such diversity are best recognised, valued and mobilised through person centred, experiential approaches to learning.
- Change, as well as being exciting and stimulating, can be a difficult and painful process.
- Effective leaders are able to influence local and national policy agendas and respond creatively in complex environments of rapid and frequent change.
- For leadership initiatives to be effective they need to be supported at all levels in the organisation.

The ways in which the RCN Clinical Leadership Team work are underpinned by a shared understanding and commitment to the values outlined above and are expressed through:

- Keeping the provision of excellent evidence-based patient/client care central to the Programmes.
- Working in partnership with organisations to develop individuals within the workplace.
- A commitment to the professional and personal development of individual participants through the use of experiential learning methods, personal development plans and needs led workshops.
- A focus on the clinical and organisational context within which health and social care is delivered.
- The development of a culture congruent with our values, within the Clinical Leadership team itself and the wider RCN; within the Programmes; with our external relations and in our partnerships (see Figure 7.1).

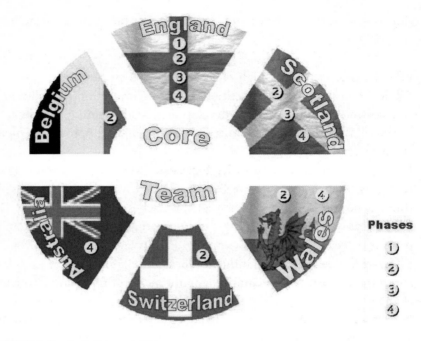

©RCN Clinical Leadership Programme 2004

Figure 7.1: Spread of the RCN Clinical Leadership Programme 1994–2003

Aims, objectives and expected outcomes

The RCN Clinical Leadership Programme is an 18-month leadership development programme which aims to assist healthcare practitioners and their teams to develop patient-centred and evidence-based strategies within the context of their day-to-day practice, organisational climate and policy agenda. In this way, the Programme impacts on individuals (patients and Clinical Leaders), teams, organisations and on policy.

The objectives of the Programme are to:

- Demonstrate improvements to patient care
- Demonstrate patient-focused approaches to organising care
- Demonstrate evidence-based practice development
- Demonstrate improvements to the learning environment and enhanced job satisfaction

- Evaluate the impact of the Programme on the leadership behaviours of the participants and the Local Facilitators
- Prepare Local Facilitators to be able to run the Programme in their own organisation after completing the initial Programme
- Enable support systems to be put in place to ensure continuation of the Programme across the NHS after completion of this initial programme of work.

Establishing the Programme

There are a number of stages to establishing the Programme. Firstly, organisations volunteer to participate. This involves liaising with the Executive Teams of NHS Trusts and ensuring that there is clarity about the Programme, including the support required and how this articulates with the organisation's leadership strategy. Once the Trusts have decided to participate, each is paired within a close geographical area for support, networking and collaboration in running workshops. This strategy has proved to be extremely effective in the Programme to date. Active participation of the Trust Board and the Director of Nursing have also been shown to be key in determining the overall success of the Programme and in maximising the impact of the Programme at every level of the organisation. Trust Boards need to demonstrate commitment to implementing organisation-wide actions that emerge from the Programme interventions as illustrated in Figure 7.2.

Having made the decision to initiate the Programme, the organisation appoints a Local Facilitator to run the Programme and support the Clinical Leaders.

Facilitation is seen as an integral part of leadership development, one of the key strengths of the Programme is that the Local Facilitator is simultaneously a participant and a facilitator, learning about self and about how to facilitate the Programme. Each of the Local Facilitators has a considerable amount of experiential learning opportunities to develop their role as facilitator. In turn, they become very strong role models to the Clinical Leaders and to their teams participating in the Programme.

One of the first priorities for the newly-appointed Local Facilitator is to establish a steering group. The steering group consists of key stakeholders (including patient representatives) and provides support and

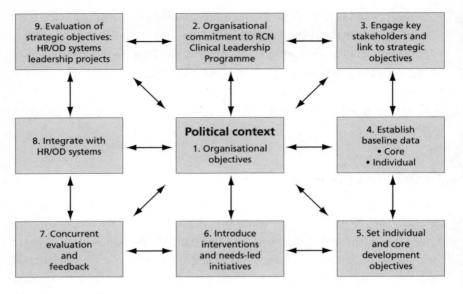

@RCN Clinical Leadership Programme 2001

Figure 7.2: Integrating the Programme into the organisation

challenge around the Programme within the organisation, including how the Programme links with the overall strategic direction of the organisation.

In the next stage of establishing the Programme, Clinical Leaders are invited to apply to participate in the Programme. Previous experience demonstrates that the preferred approach involves an open invitation to attend an overview presentation of the Programme, followed by a request for applications from Clinical Leaders who meet the following eligibility criteria:

- Voluntarily want to participate in the Programme
- Able to commit 25% of their time to the Programme over a 12-month period.

Twelve Clinical Leaders are then randomly selected from the applications received. The process is co-ordinated by the Trust. The Clinical Leaders then commence their 12-month Programme by completing a number of baseline tools and experiencing a number of other interventions, which are described below. At the end of the Programme the Clinical Leaders repeat the baseline tools and the programme is evaluated and the results are disseminated. The last two stages of interventions and evaluation are now described in more detail.

Interventions

The following interventions are used on the programme to support the Clinical Leaders' development around the five themes of the Clinical Leadership Framework (RCN, 1997) (see Figure 7.3).

Baseline tools

The purpose of the initial data-collection is to establish a baseline of the Clinical Leader's perception of their leadership behaviour; the quality of care in their area; the context in which they are working, and the perception of the team and their manager. It also enables Programme participants to identify strengths and areas for development, providing information to construct an individual personal development plan. The personal development plans that emerge from this process are dynamic, recognising the clinical situation in which the Clinical Leader works and the need for change as new priorities emerge. The following baseline tools are used – Clinical Leader Profile, Learning Styles Questionnaire and Values Clarification Exercise. Participants also receive 360° leadership feedback.

360° leadership feedback

The Programme uses a 360° leadership feedback tool developed by Kouzes and Posner (1997). Kouzes and Posner developed the Leadership Practices Inventory (LPI) through a triangulation of qualitative and quantitative research methods and studies. In-depth interviews and written case studies from people's personal best leadership experiences generated the conceptual framework, which consists of five key or exemplary leadership practices.

• Challenging the process

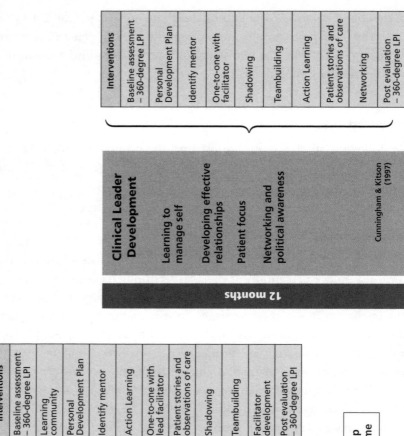

Figure 7.3: Clinical leadership framework

- Inspiring a shared vision
- Enabling others to act
- Modelling the way
- Encouraging the heart.

At the outset of the Programme the participants, their line managers, co-workers and direct reports complete the LPI. Feedback to participants is given face-to-face by the facilitator, enabling the participants to identify areas of strength and areas for development that feed into their personal development plans. The LPI is completed again at the end of the programme. Participants are then able to identify changes in their leadership behaviours and review their personal development plan for the future.

Personal development

Personal development is an integral part of the Clinical Leadership Programme. Personal development is seen as a crucial to the development of leaders. The Programme provides a number of opportunities for participants to develop personally. Following the 360° leadership feedback, each participant creates a personal development plan and identifies areas of strength and areas for development. The following interventions also contribute to the participant's personal development.

One-to-ones

Each participant on the Programme has at least an hourly one-to-one every four or six weeks – the Clinical Leader with the Local Facilitator and the Local Facilitator with an RCN Facilitator. The purpose of the one-to-one sessions is to explore how the participants are experiencing the Programme, whether they are managing their time to participate effectively and to provide an opportunity for further challenge and support which contributes to their personal development.

Mentoring

Each participant of the Programme is encouraged to find a local mentor once they have received their 360° feedback. The role of the mentor is to assist the Clinical Leader and Local Facilitator and to offer a strong leadership role-model to work closely with the participant throughout the Programme. Mentors provide good networking and political opportunities. Participants are encouraged to choose carefully and have found both Trust Board members and individuals external to their organisations extremely valuable.

Shadowing

Clinical Leaders and Facilitators are encouraged to consider who they could shadow who would enable them to develop their leadership potential. Usually the participants choose somebody who they admire for their leadership qualities or somebody they want to learn more about and to understand their way of working. Ultimately the participants need to consider how the shadowing experience will contribute to their leadership development.

Action Learning

Action Learning is an 'action approach to learning', enabling personal, professional, managerial and organisational development. It is based on the belief that the most effective learning takes place in the context in which people are working. Action Learning is a key process for learning from experience, by questioning, challenging, supporting and reflecting with others on experiences to gain further insight, to agree actions and to learn from the actions taken.

Every participant on the Programme is in an Action Learning set and each Action Learning set has a facilitator.

Team-building

Clinical Leaders and Facilitators on the Programme are also enabled to develop creative ways of developing their teams. A number of team-building techniques are introduced to help establish how a group of individuals work together; how the strengths and areas for development of individuals contribute to joint working, and how groups can be helped to work more effectively as a team to achieve their primary task.

Observation of care/practice

Observation of care/practice is a simple quality improvement and personal development tool that holds an important message: that 'seeing' and 'observing' are not the same. We often take for granted what we see around us, particularly when we are busy. The approach to observation of care on the Programme was created from the original piece of action research on the programme (RCN, 1997). The approach involves two observers – an insider and an outsider. The Clinical Leader (insider) and an outsider (either the Local Facilitator or another Clinical Leader) observe and record the insider's clinical area for 30 minutes. Both the observers then share what they observed and recorded, always starting with the insider. They then conduct a critical dialogue about what they observed. The observers then share their observations with the other clinical staff who were present at the time of the observation. Areas for improvement are identified, action agreed and good practice celebrated. The Clinical Leaders, with the support of the Local Facilitators and steering group, implement and monitor the agreed actions.

Patient/client/carer stories

Patient stories (also known as patient narratives) are audio-taped interviews with patients about their experience of being in hospital or of receiving care in other settings. This is a powerful way of getting patients to help identify areas for quality improvement and to find out which aspects of their experience they value. Clinical Leaders pair up with each other to ensure that they do not do any of the patient stories in the area that they work. Patients are randomly selected and invited to tell their story about their experience of receiving patient care. The stories are audio-taped, and mind-mapped. The tape and mind-map is then given to the other paired Clinical Leader to verify. Once six stories have been collected from one clinical area, the Clinical Leaders theme the stories to identify the areas that patients did and did not value. The themes are then fed back to the multi-disciplinary team, so that areas for improvement can be identified. Action plans are then agreed and implemented. The Clinical Leaders, with the support of the Local Facilitators and steering group, again implement and monitor the agreed actions.

Intervention and needs-led workshops

The programme includes a number of intervention workshops including:

- Personal development
- Action Learning
- Team-building
- Patient stories and observations of care
- Networking and political awareness.

Needs-led workshops are also included, and while these vary between organisations they commonly include input around such areas as conflict management, dealing with difficult situations and influencing skills.

Evaluation

Evaluation of the Programme is both formative and summative. Throughout the Programme evaluations from Action Learning sets and workshops, as well as feedback from the participants, shapes the Programme, ensuring that it is needs-led to support the participants – taking account of their day-to-day, lived-in experience.

As mentioned earlier, at the end of the Programme participants receive another 360º leadership review. In addition to this quantitative data, during the 12-month Programme participants gather a great deal of information and evidence that traces their experience. This includes:

- Baseline tools
- Reflective diary notes
- Notes from mentor meetings, one-to-one coaching, shadowing experiences and objective-setting
- Personal development plan
- Actions and evaluation forms from Action Learning sets

- Evaluation forms and notes from workshops
- Review of updated action plans from patient stories and from observations of care.

In the spirit of adult learning, this evidence belongs to the participants. However, the Clinical Leaders are encouraged to use this evidence to reflect on their learning over the twelve months. Using trigger questions, themes are identified by the Local Facilitator that captures the Clinical Leaders' experiences. In addition to this data, the Programme is also evaluated locally by looking at the action plans from patient stories and observations of care and by undertaking focus groups with key stakeholders, such as Directors of Nursing and other members of the Executive Team, mentors and team members. The Programme outcomes are then disseminated at local conferences which tend to be organised and led by the Clinical Leaders.

Programme impact

This section focuses on how the Programme works with Local Facilitators and Clinical Leaders to ensure that they are able to articulate the impact of the Programme to key stakeholders. The RCN Clinical Leadership Team were struck by the number of very emotive stories about how the Programme had changed Local Facilitators and Clinical Leaders' lives and by descriptions of the Programme as one of the participants' most powerful learning experiences. The Clinical Leadership Team concluded that some participants were better able to speak about the *process* of doing the programme, as opposed to the impact.

Programme participants therefore needed some support in articulating the impact of the Programme in relation to their leadership role, patient care, their teams and the organisation. Despite evaluations demonstrating impact at all of the levels mentioned above the Clinical Leaders were not used to presenting their achievements confidently. As a result of these observations by the Clinical Leadership Team, programme participants are now facilitated not only to describe the experience of being on the Programme, but also to consider the impact of the Programme is having at an individual, team, organisation and policy level.

This can be illustrated by quotes from Programme participants about their experience and the impact of the Programme.

Impact on individuals

Clinical Leaders and Local Facilitators evaluate the Programme to be highly effective. Common themes to emerge from their evaluations are increased amounts of confidence and personal awareness; people re-energised about working within the NHS; development of a number of practical strategies to enhance the quality of patient care and a healthier work-life balance. The interventions that the Programme participants attribute these changes to are the 360° leadership feedback, the one-to-ones, mentoring and Action Learning.

The following quotes illustrate some examples of Clinical Leaders and Local Facilitator's experience of the Programme.

> "I rationalised my life and discovered who I am."
>
> Local Facilitator

> "The programme has been the most powerful learning experience I have ever had."
>
> Clinical Leader

A Clinical Leader talked about how receiving 360° leadership feedback raised her awareness and influenced her changing behaviour.

> "It has raised my awareness more. I looked at where I did not score so highly and I have tried to think about how I can actually change my behaviour in terms of trying to be more inspirational."

The interventions such as 360° leadership feedback, mentoring, one-to-ones and Action Learning provides ongoing feedback for participants. Learning to listen more is a common outcome for participants, as illustrated in the following quote:

> "I listen more to people, especially my team and as a result of listening I feel we are a much more effective team."
>
> Clinical Leader

A Clinical Leader talking about how Action Learning increased her confidence and enabled her to move issues forward with her manager:

> "The Programme has given me a lot of confidence to actually take certain projects and things forward, to be a little more assertive in what I want to do in terms of my clinical area."
>
> Clinical Leader

A Clinical Leader talking about how the Programme has made her more assertive and has resulted in her being "a doer":

> "I am more assertive, I was already an assertive person but I'm more assertive and I am actually a doer now. Well I was a doer but, a hesitant doer. I'm actually implementing ideas I have. I am actually discussing ideas I have. I notice that I share these ideas more not only with students but also with doctors and my managers. I speak more freely to the managers. I am not happy anymore to just sit with it and moan, as we tend to do. I actually take it forward and try to get something done about it."
>
> Clinical Leader

The impact of the above interventions on the participants means that they are much more proactive in their roles and feel much more in control of their clinical agendas.

Impact on the patients

Patient stories and observations of care are two interventions which provide the Programme participants with opportunities to stand back and examine how care is being experienced by patients and delivered by their teams. Participants describe both of these interventions as being very powerful at identifying areas of good practice and also areas for improvement as the following quotes illustrate:

> "I seem to have been able to have an opportunity to just stand back and interview patients, which you don't always have an opportunity to do, and ask them about what their experiences are of being in hospital."
>
> Clinical Leader, Acute Trust

"Talking to the patients was great, as I don't do a lot of talking to patients, as much as I would like to."

Clinical Leader, Mental Health Trust

Patient stories gave an opportunity for the Clinical Leaders to understand the issues that were important to patients:

"There were stories about small aspects of the care, about how there were long days and how there didn't seem to be much activity on the ward, and they were quite bored at times. They talked about the music behind the nurses' station on a couple of occasions. They talked about, that some of the staff were quite special in the things that they did for them and so identified them by name, particularly members of nursing staff."

Clinical Leader, Acute Trust

"The other thing that a patient mentioned was the noise from music behind the nurses' station and many wards have radios behind nurses' stations because it creates some background noise, but on a couple of occasions patients mentioned how annoying that the music was – and it went on all day and it never got switched off."

Clinical Leader, Acute Trust

The patient stories also highlighted areas that the Clinical Leader needed to act on to ensure quality care in their areas and areas where care was of a high standard:

"Things like, certain themes came up like noise at night;, staff not being kind – meaning sort of – if they need something they have to wait for hours before they are helped, etc. The attitude of staff – rudeness. Other themes that came up were of staff, with doctors not explaining enough. Waiting period again – sometimes the waiting period shocks you because one lady said, she actually said that she waited for three-and-a-half hours and I couldn't believe it. She actually waited on the suite for three-and-a-half hours and then ended up being sent home to come back the following day for her operation. So that really struck home to me because I guess normally we would not be aware of that unless an official complaint came through and that also takes into consideration certain things like the process involved in preparing the clients for their elective operations, etc. So that's being looking into too."

Midwife, Acute Trust

Clinical Leaders particularly valued how easy observations of care were to set up and that they provided the opportunity for Clinical Leaders to observe care and the clinical environment objectively, to improve quality of care and have good care acknowledged:

> "It actually demonstrated good care, not weak care or care that I would be concerned about. For me it was an eye-opener in that way."
>
> Intensive Care Clinical Leader, Acute Trust

> "They were quite easy to set up. It doesn't take hardly anything in terms of preparation in terms of resources. There were very little requirements there. So it is simple and straightforward and there is an immediate feedback as well. So as regards to impinging on workload it really doesn't – and that is good."
>
> Clinical Leader, Acute Trust

> "It just makes you much more aware. You just become so blasé in the area that you work in because you're there everyday and you just don't see the very fine small details that patients have to put up with."
>
> Clinical Leader, Acute Trust

> "You think you are fine, you know. Nobody does anything wrong where I work – and to take that, you know, to sit back and do obser-vations of care, you think "Oh My God", you know, do we really do that?"
>
> Clinical Leader, Acute Trust

The Clinical Leaders were able to action issues highlighted during observations of care:

> "It was things like nurses walking down the centre of the ward and not acknowledging there were patients there, just going from A to B. But I think that comes with time if you like. I can spot an IV that is on the end within a mile, I think we all can with experience and years of walking up and down a ward. Hand washing came up, the most, I think the dramatic thing and I think everybody has found this, is the noise on the wards. Whether it be in a new area, an open area the noise of the wards you can be down at the bottom of a bay and you can hear the phones, you can hear conversations, you can hear patient's names which was a bit, it's not nice. But that has been taken on board, I think everyone of us have identified that so we will go to

the Board with it en masse, you know, and we are thinking of putting doors across the bays to cut down on noise."

Clinical Leader, Acute Trust

"Because on this ward in particular there have been a team that have been together for many, many years and over the last three years the team has changed over, people still hang on to how we would have done things and I think coming into an area and saying " Oh, we have changed that" is one thing that I have ... from taking up this post but after a while it does get tiring and it is easy to not challenge as often and as frequently as you had initially for an easier life and so doing this course made me, you know, pick up issues and challenge the practice and not just challenge it, but encourage other people to challenge it."

Clinical Leader, Mental Health Trust

- In one clinical area, during a number of observations of care, all members of the health care team were seen to enter closed curtains without asking for permission. The same issue emerged as a concern for patients in their stories in that area. As a result, staff awareness resulted in velcro fastening being added to the bedside curtains – a simple and creative example of improving privacy and dignity for patients generated by the ward team.

- When a clinical leader became aware that her ward had the second highest rate of Methicillin-Resistant Staphylococcus Aureus (MRSA) infection in the hospital, she made it her goal as part of the Leadership Programme to reduce these rates. Through observations of care, she and her team identified poor handwashing techniques as the main culprit. They worked with the Infection Control Team and Clinical Governance Manager, using skills and strategies learned in the Programme. The recent audit shows that this ward now has the lowest rate of MRSA in the Trust and is the only one to have made such a marked difference.

"Throughout the programme, I have learned to challenge other professionals on my ward, particularly consultants, about poor handwashing. More importantly I learned how to transfer these skills to my staff for more effective results."

Clinical Leader

- During episodes of observations of care and patient stories a lack of pillows was noted. As a result of these findings one Trust is considering centralising all ward/department budgets for pillows and has changed the categorisation from "luxury" to an "essential" item to ensure adequate supplies.

Patient stories and observations of care are practical tools that link clearly to the policy agendas – for example, strong links have been made with the Essence of Care (Department of Health, 2001) and the NHS Quality Improvement Scotland programmes locally, ensuring combined working at a practical level to make improvements. For example:

- Water dispensers installed in special care wards where patients have no access to kitchens (West London Mental Health NHS Trust),
- Activity afternoons organised by Health Care Assistants to prevent boredom on the wards – a main theme from patient stories on a busy cardiology ward in North Tees (North Tees and Hartlepool NHS Trust),
- Local guidelines developed to help service users handle family bereavements (Surrey Oaklands NHS Trust),
- Patient diaries introduced for parents of children with special needs who go into respite care – after patient stories showed that parents wanted to know what activities their children were doing
  (Royal Liverpool Children's NHS Trust).

There is a strong emphasis at the beginning of the Programme to ensure Local Facilitators are clear about the policy agenda and how it translates to Trust Board objectives and how, in turn, to ensure that the agenda is translated in a meaningful way to Clinical Leaders.

Directors of Nursing commenting on this impact said:

> "You can see the difference in the Clinical Leaders and their teams, there is a real buzz in these wards."
>
> Director of Nursing

> "I expected a powerful impact and it has been really very powerful."
>
> Director of Nursing

"They are really taking things on, making changes at clinical level ...
basically managing much more effectively."

Director of Nursing

Conclusions and future directions

The RCN Clinical Leadership Programme is one of a number of success-ful clinical leadership programmes. The practical patient-focused and needs-led nature of the Programme which supports Clinical Leaders through complex change has captured the attention of nursing leaders and policy makers because it offers an empirically-based programme for the delivery of the policy agenda for leadership in the modernised NHS (Cunningham and Kitson, 2000). Other success factors are dependent on the organisation's ability to align and integrate the Programme to the overall organisational strategy, therefore ensuring there are structures and systems in place to support ongoing leadership development across the whole organisation.

Providing a space through protected time appears to provide Clinical Leaders with the capability to re-energise and re-focus on why they joined the Health Service in the first place – to provide quality care for patients. In turn, this enhances their personal effectiveness and ability to work cohesively in a team.

Clinical Leaders find the Programme relevant and highly user-friendly and most importantly, effective. The Clinical Leadership Team's commit-ment to ongoing refinement of the Programme also ensures a high-quality, cost-effective product. From 2000 to 2003, the Team has been develop-ing local teams of experienced facilitators who will be pivotal at ensuring the successful, and rapid roll-out of the work. The growing national and international recognition of the Programme is based on its high quality and its commitment to effective delivery processes.

Geraldine Cunningham led the original research into the Project and had through out her career believed passionately that, against all odds, nurses can make a difference to the experiences of patients. She was also driven by the belief that nursing should be patient-centred and those nurses should be involved in developing strategies for resolving practice issues. The sponsors of the Project and the RCN shared those beliefs which became increasingly important as the Project developed.

Clinical leaders of the future need to be able to establish direction and purpose, inspire and motivate their teams and perhaps most importantly, they must be able to work with others across professional and organisational boundaries. Crucially, in the NHS, leaders need to be focussed on the patient's experience and able to redesign the NHS around the needs of patients.

The qualitative evidence gathered since the RCN Clinical Leadership Programme began, illustrates the real difference made by Clinical Leaders and their teams to patient care, attributable to participating in the Programme. The Programme enables Clinical Leaders to take ownership of the patient care agenda. The Clinical Leaders of the future will need these skills in abundance if they are to make a real difference.

As the Programme expands the Clinical Leadership Team is very keen to stay focused to the original principles that underpin it. As a result of the success of the Programme, a number of new initiatives are currently being established – Clinical Team Development, Leadership at the Point of Care, a Remote and Rural Programme and bespoke leadership development programmes. We are clear that the overall Programme framework is effective and will ensure it underpins any new developments.

We believe (and it also continues to be confirmed in our evaluations of the Programme) that being very practical, patient-focused and needs-led in nature and supporting individuals through complex change appear to be the indicators for the success of the Programme.

The RCN Clinical Leadership Programme recognises that Clinical Leaders are key to delivering successful change in a modern NHS and that leadership development programmes serve best when underpinned by the following assertions:

- A belief that individuals can make a difference
- Leadership at all levels of an organisation
- Recognition that leadership development is an ongoing process – programmes and courses are a starting point
- Experientially-based programmes
- An emphasis on developing a culture where patient-centred leadership can thrive (Cunningham, 2002).

References

Alimo-Metcalfe, B. & Alban-Metcalfe, J. (2002) "Leadership: half the battle", *Health Service Journal*, Vol. 112, No. 5795, pp 26–27.

Bass, B. (1985) "The multi-factor leadership questionnaire – form 5", in *Bass and Stogdill's Handbook of Leadership: Theory, Research and Management Applications*, 3rd edition, London, NY Free Press.

Bass, B. (1990) *Bass and Stogdill's Handbook of Leadership: Theory, Research and Management Applications*. 3rd Edition, London, NY Free Press.

Bass, B. & Avolio, B. (1994) "Shatter the glass ceiling: women may make better managers", *Human Resource Management*, 33(4) pp. 549–560.

Burns, J (1978) *Leadership*, New York: Harper and Row.

Cunningham, G., Large, S., Kitson, A., Allen E., Lister, S. & Nash, S. (2002) *Summary Evaluation Report for Phase 2 of the RCN Clinical Leadership Programme*, London, Royal College of Nursing.

Cunningham G. & Kitson, A. (2000) "An evaluation of the RCN Clinical Leadership Development Programme: Part 1", *Nursing Standard*, 15(12), pp 34–37.

Cunningham G. & Kitson, A. (2000) "An evaluation of the RCN Clinical Leadership Development Programme: Part 2". *Nursing Standard*, 15(13), pp 34–40.

Cunningham, G. (2002) *The Impact of the RCN Clinical Leadership Programme*, Brighton, National Nursing Leadership Conference.

Department of Health (2001) *The Essence of Care*, London, Department of Health.

Henderson, V. (1966) *The Nature of Nursing: A Definition and its Implications for Practice, Research and Education*. New York, MacMillan.

Heron, J. (1989) *Six Category Intervention Analysis* 3rd edition, Guildford, University of Surrey.

Kitson, A., Ahmed, L., Harvey, G., Thompson, D. & Seers, K. (1996) "From research to practice: one organisation model for promoting research-based practice", *Journal of Advanced Nursing*, Vol. 28, No. 3, pp 430–440.

Kouzes, J. & Posner, B. (1997) *The Leadership Challenge*, San Francisco: Jossey-Bass.

MacKenzie, H. & Cunningham,G. (2002) *Evaluation of Phase 3 of the RCN Clinical Leadership Programme in Scotland.*Edinburgh, Royal College of Nursing, Scotland.

Menzies, I. (1970) *The Functioning of Social Systems as a Defence Against Anxiety.* Tavistock, London.

Orem, D. (1980) *Nursing Concepts of Practice*. 2nd edn., New York, McGraw-Hill.

Paplau, H. (1952) *Interpersonal Relations in Nursing: A Conceptual Frame of Reference for Psychodynamic Nursing*. NY, Putnams.

Revans, R. (1998) "The origins and growth of action learning" in Revans, R. *The ABC of Action Learning* London, Lemos and Crane.

Royal College of Nursing (1997) *RCN Ward Nursing Leadership Project – A Journey to Patient-centred Leadership,* London, RCN.

CHAPTER EIGHT

Leadership and empowerment in action

A leadership development framework for allied health professionals and healthcare scientists

Sue Smith and Fran Woodard

Clinical leadership within the NHS has, over the last decade, been afforded more attention than in previous years. There is now a clear acceptance of the linkages needed between effective leadership on the one hand and service modernisation on the other in order to gain maximal impact on front-line patient care and the reports of the Commission for Health Improvement (CHI) support this. If patients are to experience benefit from the NHS modernisation agenda, attention must be paid to clinical leadership. It is clinicians who deliver the services, so their leadership capacity and capability must be developed. Transformational leadership, empowerment and leading change through people are all areas, which are central to the delivery of high-quality patient care.

The NHS Leadership Centre commissioned the "Leading an Empowered Organisation" (LEO) programme' from the University of Leeds to support the development of clinical leaders. The National Nursing Leadership Programme (NNLP) originally commissioned LEO, with 32,050 nurses accessing the programme. The Allied Health Professions and Healthcare Scientists (AHP and HCS) programme (which is the focus of this chapter) commissioned a further 9,500 places to provide development for AHPs and HCSs across England. This has been an extremely successful project and its scope and complexity has generated much rich learning for the future.

The purpose of this chapter is to provide background to the project; to describe the programme and its expected outcomes, and to identify the learning derived – from the perspectives of the national NHS Leadership

Centre team, the University of Leeds, and the NHS facilitators and administrators. This learning is relevant and valuable to anyone setting up such a leadership programme –whether locally, regionally or nationally.

A national strategy of leadership development

The NHS Plan (DOH, 2000) highlights the importance of leadership development. The NHS Leadership Centre was established as part of the Modernisation Agency from April 2001. The objective of the Leadership Centre is "to deliver a step change in the calibre of NHS leadership." and its strategic aim is "to influence and improve the leadership of health improvement and health and social care and to support staff in delivering improved services to patients, their families and carers and to the wider community."

In order to achieve this objective, the Centre introduced to the NHS a system of development that relied on local involvement and total system integration. What follows is a description of the programme, which focussed on AHPs and HCSs.

The focus on allied health professions and healthcare sciences

The AHP and HCS leadership focus was initiated by the launch of two key publications – "Meeting The Challenge: A Strategy For Allied Health Professions" (DOH, 2000b) launched by the Minister of State for Health in November, 2000, and "Making The Change A Strategy For The Professions In Healthcare Science" (DOH, 2000c) launched by the Minister of State in February, 2001. Both these strategies clearly acknowledged leadership development as a high priority for the clinical professions concerned.

AHPs and HCSs are involved throughout many stages of the whole patient journey, and have the ability to see health services through patients' eyes. AHPs and HCSs typically work in multi-professional team settings and have a crucial role to play in reducing waiting-times, tackling key priorities and helping patients recover their independence. They are at the forefront of joined-up approaches to health and social care, working across professional and organisational boundaries to ensure appropriate access for patients in all settings. AHPs and HCSs are therefore key in leading the way forward in delivering change.

A leadership development programme

The AHP and HCS programme was designed to increase leadership capacity to deliver a modernised and responsive Health Service. The programme was designed with the key premise that AHPs and HCSs are key to the achievement of a patient-centred needs-driven NHS. A key priority of the programme was the issue of *sustainability* of leadership development and *capacity* in relation to staff retention, new ways of working and new and extended roles.

Once a National AHP and HCS Leadership Group was launched, a decision was taken to obtain national consensus on leadership values. This was achieved through a national conference held in March, 2000. AHP and HCS professional bodies, key representatives of the professions concerned and staff of the NHS Leadership Centre were all present. Other smaller events were held which included patients and other professional groups in order to endorse and formalise the outcomes from the national conference. The core leadership characteristics or values which were identified were:

- Integrity
- Communication skills
- Passion
- Insight.

Two additional clear messages arose from the conference:

1. Leadership is an issue for everyone at all levels of an organisation.
2. Leadership is essential in order to modernise the NHS.

The Chief Executive of the NHS Modernisation Agency, in launching the programme stated that:

> "The Leadership Programme for AHPs and HCSs is central to the Modernisation Agency's work and to the aims of the NHS Plan. Nurturing leadership in Allied Health Professions and Healthcare

Scientists is essential if we are to achieve real modernisation in the NHS."

The overall AHP and HCS programme took a multi-faceted approach and delivered leadership development across the many phases of professional careers from immediate and local clinical leadership to Director level.

The core development for clinical leaders was through the introduction of the three-day Leading an Empowered Organisation programme.

The LEO programme

In order to support clinical leaders in the field it was essential to institute a development programme that would achieve professional practice accountability and so improve patient care. LEO was created originally by Marie Manthey, President Emeritus of Creative Health Care Management (CHcM) in Minneapolis, USA. In the UK the programme has been developed and provided by the Centre the Development of Healthcare Policy and Practice at the University of Leeds.

The core purpose of LEO is to enable clinical leaders to become skilled in managing, leading, team-building and staff empowerment. The focus is on the leadership and empowerment of all staff in organisations to meet their goals and objectives. The aim of attendance at a LEO programme is to internalise a number of key concepts. These concepts are intended to guide participants' future thinking and leadership behaviours (Manthey, 2003).

The conceptual framework includes the following core and interrelated concepts or "building-blocks" which, when combined enable empowerment in the organisation in support of the following outcomes:

1. Personal growth and development linked to the organisation's vision, mission and purpose.
2. Efficient, productive and satisfying work environments.
3. Improved patient and staff satisfaction.
4. A system that can change to improve efficiency, safety, and effectiveness and with staff with the courage to do what is right.
5. Highly motivated staff and quality improvement.

Core concepts of LEO provide the basis of learning and include:

Articulated Expectations (AE)

A leader's responsibility is to inspire, guide, direct and utilise *others* as leaders – and to be both a leader and a follower. The concept of Articulated Expectations, relates to the need for growth and development of all staff who work in organisations. In order to achieve this, a two-way communication process is essential which considers "What I need from you." and "What you need from me." Pursuing this strategy leads to ownership of these relationships regardless of position or status. This also requires assessment of self-competency and that of others and is associated with the organisation's vision, mission and purpose. The overall goal is personal growth and development linked to the organisation's vision, mission and purpose.

Responsibility, authority and accountability (RAA)

Responsibility, authority and accountability (RAA) are the three pillars that support the empowerment process. Clarity of responsibility, authority and accountability and ownership of results enables a move away from a "victim" mentality and a culture of blaming. The goal is efficient, productive and satisfying work for all.

Inter-dependence

In order to empower, it is essential to understand how to work with others both in a team and across the organisation. This requires insight into those personal behaviours that create ineffective relationship. It requires individuals to overcome unhealthy and co-dependent behaviours of caretaking and control and to replace these with healthy behaviours of trust, mutual respect, consistent and visible support, and open and honest communication. The goal is the development of personal behaviours that lead to synergy of the whole and to improved patient and staff satisfaction.

Positive discipline/learning

Effective leadership requires risk-taking as an essential component. Individuals need to try things in new and different ways in order to achieve positive results through creativity, innovation and learning. This requires clear (and legitimate) boundaries for behaviour and performance, honouring and rewarding risk-takers; providing challenging opportunities within a person's skill-level and using positive discipline as opposed to punishment. The leadership responsibility is to create an environment of learning and of systems to support learning, which result in superior performance and a reduction in errors. The goal is to make the system change to improve efficiency, safety, and effectiveness and to have the courage to do what is right.

Dialogue/consensus

Empowerment occurs when dialogue and consensus leads to decisions and actions that involve mutual investment, resulting in highly-motivated staff and quality improvement. Organisations can spend inordinate amounts of time processing problems with the wrong people using the wrong methodology.

It requires a systematic approach to problem-solving, based on having collective opinion and coming to an agreement (consensus) through openness. This includes finding new options that are not even imagined (dialogue). The goal is to have highly-motivated staff and quality improvement.

A process for achieving culture change

The plan was to achieve a "critical mass" of clinical leaders who would attend LEO and internalise these concepts and thus begin to change their behaviour to improve patient care and working lives. To achieve critical mass it was necessary to train people within their (then) local regions to deliver the LEO programme. It was also necessary to provide these individuals with further leadership development, as they needed to be role models of effective leadership in order to achieve credibility and sustainability.

Phase One

The first group of clinical leaders to attend the national LEO programme were front-line F and G grade nurses. Phase One had thus commenced in August 1999. Ten facilitators were appointed from each of the then NHS regions in England and their goal was to deliver programmes between January, 2000 and September, 2003, providing 32,050 places for F and G grades. Eighty facilitators provided this first phase of delivery. The evaluation of the programme was extremely positive (Werrett *et al.*, 2002; Woolnough & Faugier, 2002; CDHPP, 2003) and as a result a further 9,500 places were commissioned for AHPs and HCSs.

Phase Two

In November 2001, sixty facilitators from the Allied Health Professions and Healthcare Scientists were appointed and worked alongside the Nursing facilitators to share learning and expertise.

National delivery through NHS structures – AHP and HCS infrastructure models

The leadership leads and their deputies adopted a de-centralised approach to the identification and appointment of the LEO facilitators who were to be trained and locally deliver the LEO programmes. The selection was the sole responsibility of local AHP and HCS leads across the regions of the NHS in England. The potential facilitators were required to have at least three years experience of management in health and/or social care; to have a first degree or equivalent and be supported by senior management in their own organisation, who would vouch for their skills as facilitators.

Work-based learning experience

There is a stereotypical assumption that learning in a university setting is achieved through formal teaching in a classroom and is followed by some form of assessment and accreditation. We also know, however, that most learning for clinical leaders takes place outside the classroom – in practice. For this reason the learning strategy needed to encompass formal teaching, experiential activity and periods of reflection and action. Learners of clinical leadership and empowerment need to have the opportunity to be with colleagues in similar roles and settings and needed to have opportunities to talk about their own unique clinical experience of leadership to achieve true knowledge transfer.

Designing a robust programme

The design principles were based on knowledge transfer models (Davies *et al.*, 2003), and included the fostering of innovation and growth through self-discovery; stretching learners in supportive ways and encouraging self-reflection, self-assessment and the application of empowerment theory in practice. All the research papers written on leadership and empowerment are wasted if practitioners cannot apply the theory to practice.

The constraints on the design process were principally the number of days made available in the formal contract for the work and the time availability of the facilitators. All the facilitators had full-time posts and the time, which they had available to facilitate the LEO programme and for their own associated personal development was limited to a maximum of six days per month, over the period of the project (eighteen months). The design strategy focused on four areas of learning.

1. *Learning to facilitate the LEO programme* through the training of facilitators in a five-day "train the trainer" programme, followed by coaching and mentorship from both Associates of the University of Leeds and Nurse LEO facilitators who had been trained in the first phase, as well as by advanced facilitation workshops and master-classes.

2. *Learning to reflect and challenge assumptions*, through Action Learning sets.

3. *Learning about each person's personal approach to leadership* through 360° feedback, in a development centre setting by the application of a diagnostic instrument – Leadership Effectiveness Analysis (LEA)™

4. *Learning about creativity and innovation* through creative thinking, speed-reading, and memory and mind-mapping workshops.

Learning to facilitate the LEO programme

The sixty identified AHPs/HCSs attended a five-day training programme in Leeds. This provided ample opportunity for sharing best practice and learning from others. A consultant from Creative Health Care Management, Minneapolis, USA facilitated the programme, supported by members of the CDHPP team. The programme content included formal classroom teaching methods of key concepts; group work and opportunity to practice their newly acquired skills.

As each facilitator ran their first two LEO programmes, they were supported by experienced facilitators and Associates of the university who were also responsible for agreeing their competence on the their third programme. They then delivered a minimum of ten programmes each over the next eighteen months.

Learning to reflect and challenge assumptions

There were eight cohorts of facilitators (sixty in total) – one cohort from each of the then eight regions in the NHS in England. Each cohort attended a maximum of three Action Learning sets and also met as a learning group together with local administrators and AHP/HCS leads.

Action Learning is based on the belief that learning is made up of both programmed knowledge (traditional instruction) plus questioning insight (or critical reflection). The originator of Action Learning suggests that the best way to address on ones' own difficult problem is to help someone with his or hers (Revans, 1998). It was essential that the facilitators had such a forum to share their experience of facilitating the programme with like-minded peers who, in turn, would provide critique and thus a means of developing new skills and practice. The Action Learning sets also provided a forum for developing action plans in relation to the facilitators' personal development, teamwork and managing the system of roll-out of the programme.

Learning about one's personal approach to leadership

In order to be an effective facilitator of LEO, it is essential to be able to model rather than mould the new behaviours. It was important for the facilitators to develop an awareness of their unique personal approach to leadership. In order to enable this awareness, a two-day development centre was designed by the University of Leeds, which provided the opportunity for the facilitators to receive feedback on their approach to leadership from their immediate boss, their peers and their direct reports. An internationally-respected diagnostic Leadership Effectiveness Analysis (LEA)™ was used. It is designed to highlight potential individual assets and liabilities vis-à-vis each person's approach to leadership. It supports those using it to identify and implement specific development strategies.

The format of the feedback is derived from three areas of diagnosis; a self-completed questionnaire, nine observer questionnaires (one boss, four peers and four direct reports). Feedback is provided in the forms of:

Resource guide booklet

This has extensive interpretive information on twenty-two leadership practices, clustered in six functions of leadership (creating a vision, developing followers, implementing the vision, following through, achieving results and team playing).

One-to-one coaching

Feedback is given in a comprehensive text format and is supported by one-to-one coaching. It is presented visually, showing the degree to which the leader uses the behaviour as compared to a UK normative group and how this is impacting on the leader's approach. Concrete and tangible action steps to strengthen and improve relationships with boss, peer and direct reports are also included in the feedback.

Group support and keynote speakers

The development centre approach also included keynote speakers to set the scene in relation to the national AHP/HCS leadership activity across the country. All the events were residential to provide time and opportunity for socialising and creating new personal and professional networks. This was considered to be vital for the sharing of best practice both for the present and the future.

Learning about creativity and innovation

In a complex healthcare system like the NHS, it is vital that leaders are able to keep up with a regular flow of information and to handle complex problem solving. For this reason the facilitators identified the skills of creative thinking, memory and mind-mapping as essential components for their development. The University of Leeds (CDHPP) team provided two-day workshops related to these themes.

Evaluation of the programme impact

There are a number of studies, which provide evidence of success of the LEO programme. Some studies focus on participant reactions after the programme (CDHPP, 2003) while others focus on learning, behaviour and outcomes (Faugier & Woolnough, 2003; Werrett et al., 2002 and Cooper, 2003).

Due to the relative "recency" of LEO programmes there is currently no evidence to show change over time and therefore it is difficult to assess the degree of culture change experienced in organisations at this early stage.

Overall rating of the programme

Reaction-level data from the University of Leeds evaluation forms (CDHPP, 2003) completed by participants immediately after the programme from over 40,000 participants indicate overall general satisfaction with the LEO programme. There is evidence that participants find the programme to be valuable in preparing them for leadership and management and in helping them to appreciate the skills required to be an effective leader, manager and team player.

On average the facilitators of the programme consistently receive average scores of 4.5 out of a maximum score of 5, as does the programme rating. Qualitative analysis of the comments indicates the value participants are placing on the programme.

Faugier and Woolnough (2003) noted that, in a random sample of 109 participants who had completed feedback forms, when asked to rate the programme as: Very Good, Good, Average or Poor, 64 (or 58.7%) gave ratings of Very Good, 30 (27.5%) rated the programme as Good, 10 (9.2%) as Average and 5 (4.6%) as Poor.

Aspects relating to behaviour and attitude change

Woolnough and Faugier (2002) note that the parts of the LEO programme, which had most impact, were learning about leadership style, networking with other disciplines and a realisation that the problems faced were not unique. The kinds of changes which participants reported in their behaviour included the use of more directive behaviours; communicating more assertively; delegating more (and giving more responsibility to others rather than overloading themselves); recognising and valuing differences in leadership styles and an increase in personal awareness.

Aspects linked to improvement in patient care

When asked whether LEO had impacted on patient care, Faugier and Woolnough (2002) report that some participants immediately made the link by stating that after attendance at LEO, they encouraged patients to provide some levels of care for themselves, indicating an appreciation of patient empowerment. Others found it difficult to make the connection because they had perceived the LEO programme to be related to working with their peers and managers in their leadership role rather than it being related to patient care. Yet some could make the connection by suggesting that any improvement in teamwork must make an impact on patient care.

Increased team performance after the programme

Cooper (2003) conducted a post-LEO programme evaluation of 21 participants for a six-month period and reported that following the programme there was a statistically significant improvement ($p = 0.016^*$) in leaders self-rating of work place performance. For example, they made clear the goals and objectives of the team, were more trusting and created more opportunities for team members. Team members supported some of these ratings and reported that their leader was better at setting and maintaining objectives and giving them challenging opportunities. Qualitative data indicated that the LEO programme had a positive impact on communication, articulation of goals, networking, assertiveness, zones of responsibility and problem-solving.

Werrett *et al.* (2002) administered a pre-test and post-test survey to 550 participants in a pre-test and 181 in the post-test. Data were collected via a structured scale on 33 dimensions of leadership. They were able to demonstrate quantifiable differences in performance measure at the post-test in aspects of practice related to team and management issues, staff support and development, creative management and assertiveness.

Less positive reports of LEO

Duffin (2001), in contrast suggests there are many Trust managers who have been sceptical about the programme. It is argued that the ideas presented in LEO are too "woolly" and not easily applied to differing cultures. Dallard, in a letter to the Nursing Times (2002) suggested "LEO insulted his intelligence" Daniel (2001) – then a Director of Nursing and now a Chief Executive – in contrast takes the view that managers in organisations are clearly seeing the value of a programme that has been tried and tested. She indicates the LEO programme is helping to create leaders who have the maturity not to be threatened by the political and managerial agendas.

Quotes and stories

Stories and personal quotes also enhance appreciation of the programme. The following taken from evaluation forms reflect the internalisation of many of the concepts of the programme.

A few people found the "sphere of influence" idea very useful. They intend to focus their energy on only what they can change in the future

Others said they were definitely going to use Articulated Expectations with other colleagues.

"The Senior Management Team has used the LEO principles to review our decision-making processes. While we admit (openly and honestly) that this still requires work, everyone included feels enabled to continue working through the issues to get it right! We want a consensus decision!"

"Within the Senior Management Team we consciously try to use the principles of Relationship Management and this has led to more honest, open and therefore productive relationships between us."

"I don't take as much work home as I used to. Home time is for my family. LEO has brought balance into my life."

"Improved communication skills and better understanding of how to lead and manage people."

"The course did change my way of thinking and interacting with other people."

"More assertive and confident. I understand situations more clearly."

"I feel more confident to verbalise my expectations. I am less intimidated by other professionals."

"Confidence-boost. Have learnt some new tricks which work!"

"Top ten tips": learning from the perspectives of the national team, the University of Leeds, facilitators and administrators

Many organisations came together to ensure the success of the national leadership development programme for AHPs and HCSs. Learning from the experience and sharing that learning is an important aspect of effective leadership. Ten 'top tip' statements follow that reflect aspects of learning that have emerged from reflections on those things that were done well and on things done less well. These top ten areas of learning would be of interest to others considering creating a national programme.

1. Ensure that the administration system is decentralised sufficiently to ensure local ownership.

2. Focus on multi-disciplinary involvement at every level in order to promote sharing of best practice.

3. Establish a national data-base system that is inter-linked and compatible with local networks.

4. Insist on well-trained project managers, both locally and nationally.

5. Initiate collaborative networks of administration and lead personnel and establish trained communication champions in all local areas to effect timely and accurate information.

6. Link the national leadership strategy to other national and local organisational strategies to promote cohesion and sustainability of vision.

7. Create systems and processes that ensure equity of uptake and foster development of both high-performing and low-performing organisations.

8. Establish a process for identifying local organisations who can provide low-cost venues and avoid changes to national infrastructures during programme roll-out, as this can cause confusion.

9. Have in place clear personnel specifications and expectation frameworks for facilitators of the programme. Ensure equitable selection interviews and arrange formal written support from senior managers for the appointment of facilitators.

10. Share best practice among the facilitators through regular networking, development programmes, master-classes and Action Learning sets.

Conclusion

In summary then, effective clinical leadership is key to delivery of the NHS Plan and the associated modernisation agenda. This means clinical staff being empowered to make a difference directly to patient care. It involves the ability to question the status quo; to empower patients and recognition that it is everyone's responsibility to design and deliver the best possible services for patients. The current focus on improving patient access, experience and outcomes offers great opportunity for effective clinical leadership. A major national effort to develop the leadership skills of AHPs and HCSs should lead to a sustained improvement in patient care and career challenges and opportunities for current and future clinical leaders.

References

CDHPP (2003) *Evaluation Summaries* (unpublished), Centre for the Development of Healthcare Policy and Practice, University of Leeds.

Cooper, S. (2003) "An evaluation of the leading an Empowered Organisation Programme", *Nursing Standard* Vol. 17 No. 24 (February).

Dallard, D. (2001) *Letter in Nursing Times*, Vol. 98, No. 15 (April 9).

Davis, D., Evans, M., Jadad, A., Perrier, L., Rath, D., Sibbald, G., Straus, S., Rappolt, S., Wowk, M. & Zwarenstein, M. (2003) "The case for knowledge translation: shortening the journey from evidence to effect", *British Medical Journal*, Vol. 327, 5th July, pp 33–36.

Daniel, J. (2001) "Modernisation means buying into a new kind of leader", *NHS Magazine* (February).

Department of Health (2000a) *The NHS Plan*, London HMSO.

Department of Health (2000b) *Meeting The Challenge: A Strategy for Allied Health Professions*, London, HMSO.

Department of Health (2000c) *Making The Change: A Strategy for the Professions in Healthcare Science*, London, HMSO.

Department of Health (2001*) Life Long Learning*, London, HMSO.

Duffin, C. (2001) "Hear LEO's roar" *Nursing Standard*, Vol. 15 No. 21, pp. 12–13, (February 7).

Faugier, J. Woolnough, H. (2002) "Blazing a trail", *Nursing Times*, Vol. 98, No. 50, pp. 23–28 (December 10).

Faugier, J. Woolnough, H. (2003) "Lessons from LEO: Part One", *Nursing Management*, Vol. 10 No. 2 (May).

Faugier, J. Woolnough, H. (2003) "Lessons from LEO: Part Two", *Nursing Management*, Vol. 10 No. (June).

Manthey, M.(2003) *LEO Facilitator Manual*, Creative Health Care Management, Minneapolis.

Revans, R. (1998) *The ABC of Action Learning*, London: Lemos & Crane.

Werrett, J., Griffiths, M.& Clifford, C. (2002) "A regional evaluation of the impact of the leading an Empowered Organisation Leadership Programme", *NT Research* Vol. 7 No. 6 pp 459–470.

Woolnough, H. Faugier, J. 2002 "An evaluative study assessing the impact of the Leading An Empowered Organisation Programme", *NT Research* Vol. 7, No. 6, pp 412–421.

CHAPTER NINE

Action Learning
A case study in supporting
Clinical Leadership Development

Linda Dack

This chapter describes as a case study the establishment of an Action Learning set as an adjunct to the LEO programme to support the development of leadership skills amongst six newly appointed Senior 1s, drawn from the Allied Health Professions. It seeks firstly to establish the context for leadership development amongst the Allied Health Professions. Secondly, it provides a description of the various components of the programme and its subsequent evaluation which is based on the words of those who have experienced Action Learning as participants. Hence it seeks to illustrate through a single case study the potential value of Action Learning from workplace problems, which may sustain and enhance leadership development.

Background and context

Across the NHS, considerable effort is being directed towards the development of leadership amongst clinical staff. This is in part responding to the NHS modernisation agenda, which calls for (amongst other things) a wider involvement of clinical staff in leadership as a means of improving and modernising care (DoH, 1997). Furthermore, there is a need to develop leadership skills as more complex roles are undertaken; whole systems working becomes more commonplace; team-working breaks down professional barriers and there is increased involvement in the leadership of Clinical Governance.

The Allied Health Professionals (AHPs) are now increasingly being grouped together, both nationally and locally. This joining-together of different professional groupings under the "umbrella" of the AHPs is in its infancy and has arguably allowed the emergence of a common voice for these professions which they previously lacked. This voice is now audible at both national and local level. Whilst not a homogenous group they do nevertheless share are a number of core skills common to all these separate individual professions.

National context

"Meeting The Challenge", a national strategy for the Allied Health Professions (DoH,2000) outlined the Government's plans for developing and supporting Allied Health Professionals to meet the needs of a modern Health Service. Within this strategy there was explicit recognition of the need to develop leadership skills amongst the Allied Health Professions by offering:

• Opportunities to develop wider leadership skills as more complex roles are undertaken
• Increased involvement in the leadership of Clinical Governance
• Development of leadership skills alongside other clinicians and managers to help break down professional barriers and to build working relationships
• Leadership development focused on whole systems working.

A National Leadership Development Programme for AHPs was subsequently developed with funding through the NHS Leadership Centre. This included a range of leadership development programmes and conferences. It is not the intention here to describe the programme in detail (this is addressed in Smith and Woodard's chapter) but its existence nevertheless indicates a growing national awareness of the importance of leadership development within the AHPs.

Local context

The setting for this case study is an integrated Allied Health Professionals Directorate which came into being on 1st April 2001, with the joining of nine separate professional groups with overall leadership provided by a Clinical Director of AHPs. This novel working arrangement brought together the AHPs from an Acute NHS Trust and a Primary Care Trust within one health economy. It also included partnerships with local authority Social Services, reflecting the joint arrangements for Occupational Therapy, which have been in place since 1984. The Allied Health Professionals Directorate incorporates Art Therapy, Audiology and Hearing Therapy, Dietetics, Occupational Therapy, Orthoptists, Orthotics, Podiatry, Physiotherapy; and Speech and Language Therapy, each under the leadership of a professional Head of Service.

Strategic leadership and overall operational responsibility rests with a Clinical Director of the service. This model of service provision arose out of a need to bring together the Allied Health Professions into one whole across the different elements of a natural health and social care community. The Directorate has over 300 staff members, both registered and non-registered practitioners. Staff work flexibly across the three organisations providing services as close to home as possible. The Clinical Director of the AHPs is future-orientated and wants to introduce change strategies that will allow measurable improvements to be made in patient care. Part of that approach is to develop leadership skills amongst all the staff members.

Leadership development within the Directorate

The overall approach within the Directorate to leadership development takes a number of strands, which have emerged over the two years to 2003. The first strand is access to the Leading an Empowered Organisation (LEO) programme, both locally where the NHS Trust delivers this under a licence, and through access to places on the national programme. To date across the Directorate, some 142 staff have been through the LEO programme and this represents 45% of the total Directorate workforce. The participants have included the Clinical Director, all the professional Heads of Service, 90% of Senior 1 (or equivalent) grades, and 20% of Senior 2s (or equivalent grades).

While the LEO programme has evaluated well locally (Lappin, 2003) and has been acknowledged to have influenced leadership behaviour positively (Perry, 2003), concern has been expressed as to the sustainability of these desirable behavioural changes.

The second strand is through the Leadership Effectiveness Analysis (LEA™) diagnostic. This resource is based on the principle of 360° assessment, which includes feedback on a number of leadership behaviours from the self, leader, peers, and direct reports. The aim of LEA is thus to increase awareness of different perceptions concerning effectiveness as a leader.

Across the Directorate, LEA has been used with the senior leadership roles (Heads of Service) and is now extending to the clinical specialists. In addition, two staff members are currently going through the RCN Clinical Leadership Programme (see Cunningham & Mackenzie's chapter), which is now being delivered within the organisation.

Hence the Allied Health Professions are in the forefront of inter-professional learning. However, whilst the spread of leadership development is not in doubt throughout the Directorate, the *sustainability* of leadership development needs careful consideration. Action Learning has been identified as a potential means of overcoming the issue of sustainability of leadership (Perry, 2003; Lappin, 2003). The remainder of this chapter is devoted to an exploration and subsequent evaluation of an Action Learning set as an adjunct to the 3-day LEO Programme.

Introduction to Action Learning

The idea of Action Learning, in its original form, incorporated both *set* and work. The *set* is a small group of people (usually 4–6) who meet regularly to work together on problems from their practice. The idea of people coming together to develop their ideas in a set was developed whilst the instigator of Action Learning, the late Professor Reg Revans was working at Cavendish laboratories, at Cambridge University in the late 1920s. Professor Revans and his colleagues would meet each week to discuss their work, supporting and challenging each other in order to explore the difficulties they were experiencing. From these early beginnings, Action Learning has evolved as a process, which has at its heart self-development. It has been used in numerous settings with a strong history in health and social care.

The problem (or conversely the opportunity!) is that Revans never defined what Action Learning is – rather he defined what it is not. There is a suggestion that it is in the application that we learn about Action Learning. Nevertheless, Revans does offer this explanation of Action Learning:

"Action learning is a means of development, intellectual, emotional or physical, that requires its subject, through responsible involvement in some real, complex and stressful problem, to achieve intended change sufficient to improve his observable behaviour henceforth in the problem field."

Revans, 1998

Here we can see that the main premise of Action Learning is that action and learning are bound together. Revans suggested that learning occurs in broadly two ways. Firstly, Programmed Learning or "P". "P" is based on traditional instruction and is generally aimed at imparting what experts already know. Secondly, there is learning derived from critical thinking or insightful questioning – "Q". "Q" is a process of exploring knowledge in practice. A popular misconception is to see "P" and "Q" as opposing factions, at war with one another. However, Revans took pains to explain that he did not reject "P", although he was often critical of it. He instead wanted to put it in its appropriate place in the learning spectrum and suggested that learning is based on the interaction between "P" and "Q". This observation allowed him to formulate the equation: L= P+Q. He gives further insight into the relationship between P and Q within learning when he points out that behaviour change (which many regard as being indicative of learning) is more likely to occur as a result of reflecting on experience and that questioning insight contributes to that process. Hence, reflection with others in the set affords an enriched practical learning experience. Revans further suggests that Action Learning is the Aristotelian manifestation of *work*: We learn as we do, and furthermore we do because we have learned. The question remains – do we always learn as we do? Thus one added ingredient essential for Action Learning is a conversion of "action content" into a "learning context" (Botham, 1994).

The development programme

The idea of leadership development for newly-appointed Senior 1s arose from a belief that this would support the transition into this clinical leadership role and test-out the value of Action Learning in the context of leadership development. The programme consisted of a number of elements. Firstly, access to the 3-day LEO programme being provided locally for Nurses and AHPs. Secondly, through a resource pack based upon elements of leadership development. Thirdly, through the delivery of nine monthly Action Learning set meetings of a half-day duration. Professional Heads of Service nominated willing participants who wished to engage with this approach and supported their access to the programme. Hence participation was voluntary but targeted. The participants were drawn from Physiotherapy, Occupational Therapy, Speech and Language Therapy and Audiology. The seven participants were all newly-appointed Senior 1s or equivalent grades. By the end of the programme four participants remained; two had left the organisation and a further one could not make a sustained commitment. The participants were also encouraged to keep a learning log which, although the contents would not be shared, would not only promote the concept of reflective learning but also provide a trigger for reflection and action.

The first set meeting

The first set meeting as well as introducing participants to the process of Action Learning also involved working to establish ground rules for our behaviours in the set. Whilst set procedures naturally develop over time, some initial emphasis was on the establishment of ground rules, which were concerned with: safety as in maintaining confidentiality; time keeping and attendance; participation; and the use of questioning and challenges. This laid down the foundations of the learning set. Safety was a particular important issue within the set. In addition participants were asked to choose the content of each set meeting. This was felt to provide a theme for learning from practice until the process of Action Learning was more fully established. A book entitled "A Manager's Guide To Self-Development" (Pedler, Burgoyne & Boydell, 2001) was given to participants from which they chose the theme for the set meeting. With this learning resource there are over fifty potential available themes from which to choose. The chosen themes included: understanding your learning processes; career/life planning activity; managing your time; and decision-making.

The second set meeting

A self assessment learning styles questionnaire was used in the second set meeting to assist individual set members to identify from one of four defined learning styles their individual preference. Honey & Mumford (1992) who developed this tool suggest that it is possible to develop and build one's learning styles and point out the advantages of being a conscious learner from experience. This provided a useful tool to explore the learning context from action.

Subsequent set meetings

At subsequent set meetings, time was spent on a theme and more attention began to focus on problems from practice. This is the essence of action learning when we seek greater understanding from learning from our experiences. Thus the principal focus of development becomes a work-based issue connected with the individuals' leadership development. The time was divided equally between the set members, although this time allocation could be subject to negotiation and changed if it was thought to be necessary. Some of the LEO material was revisited in particular, the problem-solving model and aspects of relationship management at the request of the participants.

Evaluation

The set explored first as a group, the impact of the set experience. Each member of the set had kept an individual reflective log and from this they each wrote a short account of their experiences. In addition, one-to-one interviews were also held with the remaining participants. As a set adviser I made notes of my own reflections of the process and shared these with the participants.

Initial expectations

Initially expectations of the programme fell into an overarching theme of "development". The following extracts from participant reflections illustrate this theme.

"Many of the essential qualities that are required to be a good team leader are never fully developed at a more junior level. I felt as a newly-appointed senior one that some elements of my role were beyond my capabilities as I had never had to deal with difficult and inappropriate behaviour from staff and found these challenging situations quite threatening."

"Although I did not know what to expect, I felt it would provide me with an opportunity to listen to suggestions and gather ideas on how to develop myself through reflection."

"As a group we identified key areas we felt were essential to develop and we also had the opportunity to work through specific problems we had encountered at work."

"I feel the self development programme has made a significant contribution to my personal development."

Outcomes

Problem-solving

Participants have learned that dialogue with others can help to reflect on problems solving and take action.

"Each member of the group had a specific problem that they wanted to discuss and therefore gave the opportunity to problem-solve different issues."

"I feel it has improved my skills to problem solve and prioritise problems."

"Personally I feel that I gained most by discussing an ongoing problem at work for me. By using a problem-solving approach, this allowed me to realise that I had more options available than I realised. By discussing the problem with the group it allowed me to be more objective about the problem and try out different ways of tackling it."

"Each member of the group had a specific problem that they wanted to discuss and therefore gave the opportunity to problem-solve different issues."

Support

The word "support" was used most by the participants to describe their experience of action learning:

> "The group members offered excellent support. I learnt a lot from other members' problems and from each individual's contribution and advice."

> "The forum of the set was always supportive and honest and encouraged sharing and problem-solving in a non-threatening manner. As the group developed, it became protected time away from the clinical area to consolidate these essential skills and our network extended to outside this forum, where we would often share problems and ask advice of each other as situations arose."

Confidence

All of the participants identified their increase in confidence as a result of the programme:

Throughout the last nine months of attending the Action Learning set, I feel that my confidence in acknowledging difficult behaviours and dealing with them appropriately has grown considerably."

> "Increased confidence to voice opinion."

> "Above all, the Action Learning set has provided me with increased confidence in my own abilities as a team leader and allowed me to realise my own strengths and weaknesses to a far greater extent."

Furthermore this increased confidence has become visible in their ability to lead and develop others:

> "I feel that this has had a positive impact on the rest of my team who feel fully supported, both personally and professionally and I have been able to help them develop some of the skills I have learned, particularly in dealing with challenging and difficult behaviour and time management."

Networking

The idea of establishing networks was considered an important outcome of the set experience:

> "I have also forged closer links with a group of peers and know that we will continue to support each other outside of this group, which will enable us to develop and learn from each other's experiences."

> "I still share ideas and run problems by two members of the group and have found this to be a support."

Here the end of a programme of Action Learning does not necessarily mean the end of an Action Learning set. Many sets continue to meet afterwards, sometimes for years afterwards. The success of an Action Learning set can probably best be judged by whether the participants continue to meet as a self-facilitating set.

Dealing with unhealthy behaviours

A key theme of the set was learning how to deal with unhealthy behaviours both in ourselves and in others:

> "I have implemented the aspects on how to handle unhealthy behaviours and killer phrases to some success, which in the past I may have chosen not to tackle. I am a confident approachable clinical however, the skills that I have taken from these groups have allowed for assertive but non-aggressive responses from myself in certain situations. Also I find I can read peoples' personality a lot better, whether they are an exploder or enjoy confrontation, this prepares myself for the responses I shall use."

> "Throughout the last nine months of attending the Action Learning set, I feel that my confidence in acknowledging difficult behaviours and dealing with them appropriately has grown considerably."

Conclusions

Whilst in its infancy, the idea of an Action Learning set to support leadership development as an adjunct to the LEO programme appears to add value. It also seems to reflect Cusins (1996) view of Action Learning which treats it as a syndrome of four mutually-reinforcing activities for creative decision-making:

- Experiential learning
- Creative problem-solving
- Acquisition of relevant knowledge
- Co-learner group support.

Naturally there are a number of lessons to be carried forward to the design of other programmes. Firstly, in the formation of the group it was important to gain support from the participants' leaders. This, amongst other things allowed them the time to participate and to ensure that leadership development was an integral part of their development plans. Secondly, moving from a taught to an untaught programme was gradual. This may have reflected my own nervousness about the transition and the time it takes for sets to become established as the vehicle for learning from actions. However, it may be the set as the learning context for leadership development is enough.

Finally, there are the resources that would be needed to roll-out this approach post-LEO for others, which may be quite extensive. However targeting individuals who are new to the leadership role may provide an opportunity to build for the future.

Whilst this is a small study, it has highlighted the value of Action Learning as an adjunct to the LEO programme.

References

Botham, D. (1994) *Ways of Thinking About Action Learning* Revans Institute for Action Learning & Research, University of Salford.

Cusins, P. (1996) "Action Learning revisited: employee counselling today", *Journal of Workplace Learning* Vol. 8, No. 6, pp. 19–26.

Department of Health (1997) *The New NHS: Modern: Dependable,* London, HMSO.

Department of Health (2000) *Meeting The Challenge: A Strategy for Allied Health Professions* London, Crown Publishing.

Honey, P. & Mumford, A. (1992) *The Manual of Learning Styles,* Maidenhead, Peter Honey Publications

Lappin, M. (2003) *Do Staff Who Have Undertaken the LEO Programme Require Further Support to Sustain and Develop Their Leadership Behaviours?*, MSc Dissertation, University of Salford.

Pedler M., Burgoyne, J. & Boydell, T. (2001) *A Manager's Guide to Self-Development* (4th Edition), London, McGraw-Hill.

Perry S. (2003) *An Exploration of Evidence of Perceived Behavioural Changes in Participants Following Accessing a Three-Day LEO Programme* – Evaluation Study, University of Salford.

Revans, R. (1998) *ABC of Action Learning,* London, Lemos & Crane.

CHAPTER TEN

Strategic approaches to Clinical Leadership Development: do they work?

Maggie Griffiths, Collette Clifford and Julie Werrett

This chapter will explore aspects of leadership development in the context of health care in the UK today The specific focus will be to examine aspects of the introduction of the Leading an Empowered Organisation (LEO) programme in the West Midland region of England in 2001.

The chapter will examine the policy development that led to the programme being introduced and some of the local issues related to that introduction. The limitations and benefits of these types of approaches will then be explored, followed by reflections on some of the themes raised.

Indira Ghandi once reflected:

"I suppose leadership at one time meant muscles; but today it means getting along with people";

or as the former Managing Director of Toshiba Computer Systems, Alan Thompson noted:

"Management is mechanical – it's about resource allocation, efficiency, optimisation...and there are processes you can follow to help you manage effectively. Leadership is different – it's about vision and fire and winning people's hearts as well as their minds'

Lucas, 2000

Although neither of these quotes was about health care, it could be argued that they are relevant to the changes that are going on currently in the NHS. The days when health care professionals, of whatever discipline, were the "muscles" is declining. Participation and collaboration are increasingly important, for example with the introduction of clinical networks. Evidence is now beginning to emerge that effective teamwork is important both in staff recruitment and retention and in patient outcomes and mortality, (West 2002, Borrill *et al.*, 2001).

Various strategies have been used to develop leaders in the public and private sectors. These range from formal taught courses, self-development and "how to do it" books, plus a variety of informal courses which help people to examine their leadership behaviours. The literature in this area shows that there is no "one best way" of developing leaders -it depends on the situations, personalities and the cultures of organisations. More information on the different styles of leadership theory can be found in Mullins, 2002. He describes leadership theories as falling into six main categories. They are the *trait or qualities* approach, the *functional or group* approach, leadership as a *behavioural category*, *styles* of leadership, the *situational* approach and *contingency* models and *transformational leadership*. The differences between leadership and management have also been widely discussed, but as Chambers (2003) notes some of these arguments now need to be put aside, and the time has come for nursing and nursing leaders to "just do it"!

Leadership development in the NHS

Before looking at the leadership strategy in more detail it is important to examine briefly the NHS Plan and why leadership development is so important to its success. In 1997 "The New NHS: Modern: Dependable" (DoH, 1997) was published followed by "A First Class Service: Quality in the NHS" (DoH, 1998). The NHS Plan (DoH, 2000a) built on these earlier documents and outlined a 10-year modernisation agenda for health care in England. The devolved governments of Scotland and Wales have produced their own modernisation plans (Scottish Executive, 2000, National Assembly of Wales, 2001) and a consultation paper for Northern Ireland has also been published, "Developing Better Services" (DoHSSPS, 2002).

- The English NHS Plan describes its approach as one of investment and reform with the aim of providing a 21st century health care service for patients and their carers. The public consultation identified that what

people wanted was:
- more and better paid staff using new ways of working
- reduced waiting times and high quality care centred on patients
- improvements in local hospitals and surgeries.

The NHS Plan noted that:

> "Leadership development in the NHS has always been ad hoc and incoherent … that will now change."

"Shifting The Balance Of Power: Securing Delivery" (DoH, 2001) was the programme of change, which aimed to empower front-line staff and patients as part of the implementation of the NHS Plan. It states that:

> "Front-line staff need to be in charge of front-line services and have the power to manage the local community needs – always within the context of clear national standards and a strong accountability framework."

In order to deliver the NHS Plan, the Government has increased investment in the NHS. This has led to greater numbers of staff working in the NHS and new and upgraded hospitals and GPs premises. All Primary Care Groups became Primary Care Trusts by 2004 with a subsequent growth in their roles and responsibilities. The target was to increase capacity overall. Intermediate and step-down facilities have been introduced to help relieve the pressure on beds in the acute hospital sector. A number of National Service Frameworks (NSFs) have been introduced for people with cancer, heart disease and diabetes. NSFs have also been produced for the elderly, children and people with mental health problems.

There has been investment in informatics to improve the flow of information between primary and secondary care facilities. There have also been changes to legislation with the introduction of the Health Act in 1999 and the National Health Service Reform and Health Care Professions Act of 2002. Chief Executives are responsible for systems to deliver high-quality care as well as financial probity. The rights of patients have been further strengthened with the introduction of patient advocacy services, the adoption of the Human Rights Act and strengthening of data protection so that patients can access their medical notes if they require them. Continuing professional development and life-long learning is now part of the agenda for all health care staff.

The establishment of the National Institute for Clinical Excellence (NICE) has provided up-to-date relevant information on effective treatment protocols. Monitoring of progress is now undertaken by the Commission for Health Improvement (CHI) and reports of their visits to NHS Trusts to check progress on the Clinical Governance agenda are available from their website (www.chi.nhs.uk). These initiatives are aimed at helping to develop a more open NHS where information is freely available to patients, their families and staff.

The expansion of CHI from April, 2004 will offer a further coming-together and expansion of their services. It will then become the Commission for Healthcare Audit and Inspection (CHAI) and be responsible for:

- Existing CHI work
- The National Care Standards Commission, in respect of private and voluntary healthcare
- The Audit Commission, in respect of national studies in the efficiency, effectiveness and economy of healthcare.

CHAI is also expected to take over the work of the Mental Health Act Commission. Its new functions will include providing an independent assessment of complaints, looking at public health arrangements and becoming the leading inspectorate in relation to healthcare. The legislation for these changes is part of the Health and Social Care (Community Health & Standards) Bill and is expected to receive Royal assent in late 2003.

For all these challenges and changes new ways of working are being introduced, traditional barriers are being challenged and effective leadership is crucial at all levels of organisations.

It is important to realise the scale of these changes. Dr Don Berwick, the US-based President and Chief Executive of the Institute of Healthcare Improvements (and until recently a member of the NHS Modernisation Board) was interviewed recently for the Health Services Journal. He described the pace of change and the progress that had already been made and argued that what the NHS is trying to do is larger and more complex than the transformation of any economic sector in recent history. (Dempsey, 2003). However, there are several things which need to be borne in mind when considering the modernisation agenda. They include:

1. The NHS Plan is a 10-year agenda. Change in health care takes time to achieve, as anyone who has been involved in this type of work will be aware.
2. Some of these changes are challenging to hard-worked staff who are trying to make changes and deliver a high quality service whilst meeting national and local targets and initiatives.
3. Support for the Government by medical and managerial staff is at an all-time low and "Shifting the Balance" will delay the implementation of the NHS Plan. There is a feeling that it may be one re-organisation too far. (Smith *et al.*, 2001).
4. "The demands of rapid organisational change being undertaken with limited managerial resources may divert attention from the tasks of modernising services and improving health" (Wilkin *et al.*, 2001).
5. A recent report from the National Audit Office (2003) on Clinical Governance reported that there were improvements where good systems were in place but also noted that there were issues in fully engaging staff in the strategy for Clinical Governance.

In order to implement such an ambitious plan for the NHS, effective leadership at all levels is crucial to its success. Yet there are words of warning if literature is examined from industry about the success of change programmes. The success rate of major change programmes in Fortune 1000 companies is between 20–50% (Garside 1998). One of the reasons for this is that leaders and employees often see change differently. To the former it is an opportunity – a development which may mean promotion and higher status. To the latter it may be perceived as disruptive and in health care organisations maybe seen as preventing people from providing clinical services.

However as Garside (1998) notes: "Increasingly managers and clinical professionals in health care are coming to terms with the need for carefully designed and implemented programmes for change, programmes which take into account the external world and its pressures – politicians,

professional groups and the public and the internal world of the organisation – its culture, norms and staff behaviours."

So where does this leave the leadership strategy as part of this agenda?
The leadership strategy was launched in 2001. It included the establishment of an NHS Leadership Centre, which is responsible for developing
all types of leaders in the NHS including clinical staff, as part of the
Modernisation Agency. There has been an increased number of new nurse
and therapy consultant posts as proposed in "Making A Difference"
(DoH, 1999) and "Meeting The Challenge" (DoH, 2000b) and this led
to the creation of 1,152 places on the Royal College of Nursing (RCN)
Clinical Leadership Programme and 32,050 places on the LEO training
programme. These are aimed at developing and supporting clinical practitioners and building a critical mass of people who can make change happen and lead teams of staff. They vary in length and content. The RCN
programme is longer than LEO, being originally created in 1995 with the
aim of identifying how clinical nurse leaders could improve the quality of
the care that patients received (see Cunningham and Mackenzie's chapter).

What is LEO?

The Leading an Empowered Organisation programme is a 3-day course,
designed for health care professionals from all disciplines and with differing levels of experience and expertise. The philosophy of the programme
is based on principles of respect, dignity and empowerment.

The LEO programme is run by the Centre for the Development of
Healthcare Policy and Practice (CDHPP) at the University of Leeds and
Creative Healthcare Management (CHcM) based in Minneapolis, USA
and was originally established by a nurse (Marie Manthey) who first
developed the concepts underpinning the LEO programme. The
CDHPP has worked with CHcM to ensure the programme is appropriate for leaders from diverse cultural backgrounds and organisations. It
encourages participants to examine their own behaviour as leaders and
followers in various situations and gives them the opportunities to practice different ways of learning new types of behaviour. The aims of the
programme are to improve relationship management and develop problem solving and risk taking skills. It teaches techniques to facilitate
empowerment in the workplace using a variety of teaching methods.

Senior nurses and therapists facilitated the programme, following a training programme organised by the CDHPP.

Why LEO?

The LEO model provides opportunity to help people examine what works and what doesn't work in their leadership behaviours with other people. Due to of the changing models of health care delivery increasing numbers and levels of staff will need leadership skills. In a recent research review on good global leadership practice it was noted that:

> "the review suggests that leadership development is about individual self-awareness of personal capabilities and capacity for leadership ... it is really not possible to lead others if you do not understand yourself."

> Tremblay and Dunn, 2002

This is where LEO provides an introduction of some of these approaches. It enables participants to examine their behaviours and provides practice in different ways of problem solving in a protected environment.

The local approach to the operation of the strategy

When the national leadership strategy was launched, the impact for the West Midlands NHS Executive of the LEO initiative element of the strategy was that over 4,000 clinical staff needed to have completed the programme by November 2002. This was to be achieved by planning 160 courses with approximately 25 people attending each programme.

By June 2002, the estimated number of nurses in the West Midlands Region who had attended the programme was 3,870 and the total number of allied health professionals who had attended was 314. Participants were drawn from all Acute and Primary Care Trusts in the West Midlands Region (PDQ, 2002). This, combined with those booked to complete the course between June and November 2002 showed that the target numbers would be achieved. In the West Midlands, funding was identified from the then Non-Medical Education and Training (NMET) levy to support this programme. This allocation included replacement costs for the programme facilitators and the costs for the venue and subsistence (light refreshment) of programme for the participants during the 3-day events (Werrett *et al.* 2002a). The programme was administered on behalf of the NHSE by the Partnership for Developing Quality (PDQ) under the direction of a Project Leader.

The next part of the chapter examines some of the issues when this type of Strategy is put into operation. One of the challenges of this strategy was that it was one part of the NHS Plan. Other parts of the Plan also had to be delivered. These included (as mentioned earlier) the implementation of the National Service Frameworks; reduction in waiting times in Accident & Emergency departments; action on waiting lists; the Clinical Governance agenda (including preparation for and visits from the Commission for Health Improvement) plus local quality improvement programmes.

The LEO course was mainly directed at F&G grade nurses and equivalent grades of the allied health professions, together with senior nursing and therapy staff who acted as facilitators for the programme. These staff were also involved in some of these other initiatives, so there may have been competing priorities for both staff and managers.

The implications of this approach include:

- *It was to be done.* It was protected development time for staff, which was free to organisations. It is interesting to note that although the West Midlands evaluation, Werrett *et al.* (2002b) reported that participants represented all the Acute and Primary Care Trusts in the West Midlands region, the numbers attending did not correlate to the numbers of clinical staff employed by the Trusts.

- *The initiative was a political imperative.* Whilst that maybe criticised as a top-down approach, it did help to ensure that time was allocated, funds were released to get the target group trained and a critical mass of clinical people with appropriate leadership skills were developed to meet the modernisation agenda targets. It provided development for staff and for the facilitators. It also helped people to develop networking opportunities. This was highly valued in the evaluations. Many respondents highlighted the opportunity to network with people from other parts of their own Trust and from different areas of care as the most important aspect of attending the LEO programme. They valued the opportunity to communicate with people from other disciplines and to learn from the experiences of others outside their working units

- "it was good to spend quality time with other people from the trust" (Woolnough and Faugier, 2002).Due to time constraints this is often difficult to achieve in day to day working. "One of the main reported benefits was the opportunities it created for networking in mixed teams." (Werrett *et al.*, 2002b)

- *Sustainability* has been helped by the National Nursing Leadership Project website, which has a range of e-learning activities building on some of the leadership programmes to help embed the principles and provide a forum for discussion and learning.

The limitations of this type of approach include are that there are competing priorities for clinical staff and managers and there is a danger that a "tick-box" approach may be adopted to ensure that numbers are filled rather than appropriate staff recruited. The programme was targeted at F&G grade nurses and equivalent allied health professionals. However, within nursing in the West Midland evaluation, staff attended from grades E to Senior Nurse Practitioner level (Werrett *et al.*, 2002b) and some of the negative comments from the national evaluation were from people at grade I or senior allied health professional level (Woolnough and Faugier, 2002)

Conclusion

So how does this affect the patients and their care? Does the leadership strategy and the operation of that strategy impact on patient care and the experiences of patients and their families? Will this approach modernise the NHS? As Bate (2000) notes:

> "All the evidence suggests that it is leadership above all else that makes the difference between the success of failure of a change programme. What is required is first a redefinition of leadership and second the building of a process of leadership that will deliver the modernising agenda."

Hewison (2003) states:

> "This belief that leadership can bring about transformation and deliver new ways of working is a central feature of current approaches to leadership in the NHS."

However leadership development is only part of the issue as Wilson Barnett (2003) notes "Many authors talk of leadership in a vacuum, but it would seem that appropriate actions depend on the activities, setting and resources available."

For this to happen leadership discussions need to be integrated into the debate on developing safe and effective practitioners who are open to appropriate change which improves the care given to people and their families.

Whether this type of leadership development works is under question and may not be answered until the wider question of whether the NHS Plan and the modernisation agenda has been delivered and 21st century health care is available to all. Whether the "big-bang" approach to these type of issues works is interesting to debate. Much depends on the organisational culture and where and how it fits with an organisation's overall strategy and development plan. The leadership strategy has been launched and the LEO programme is part of it as a catalyst for change. Will it work? The jury is still out!

References

Bate, P. (2000) "Leading the NHS from a different place" *Health Services Management Centre Newsletter,* School of Public Policy, University of Birmingham Vol 6 Issue 2 p.2.

Borrill, C., West, M., Dawson, J., Shapiro, D., Rees, A., Richards, A., Garrod, S., Carletta, J. & Carter, A. (2001) *Team Working and Effectiveness in Health Care,* Birmingham, Aston University.

Chambers, N. (2002) "Nursing leadership: the time has come to just do it" *Journal of Nursing Management* Vol. 10 No. 3, pp 127–128. Available from: http://dx.doi.org/10.1046/j.136.

Dempsey, P. (2003) "A case of us and them, the HSJ interview: Don Berwick" *Health Service Journal* (10 April), pp 20–21.

Department of Health (1997) *The New NHS: Modern: Dependable*, London, HMSO.

Department of Health (1998) *A First Class Service: Quality in the NHS*, London, HMSO.

Department of Health (1999) *Making a Difference: Strengthening the Nursing Midwifery and Health Visiting Contribution to Health and Healthcare*, London, DoH.

Department of Health (2000a) *The NHS Plan*, HMSO, London.

Department of Health (2000b) *Meeting the Challenge: a Strategy for Allied Health Professions,* London, HMSO.

Department of Health (2001) *Shifting the Balance of Power: Securing Delivery*, London, HMSO.

Department of Health, Social Services and Public Safety (2002) *Developing Better Services: Modernising Hospitals and Reforming Structures.* London TSO.

Garside, P. (1998) "Organisational context for quality: Lessons from the fields of organisational development and change management" *British Medical Journal* Quality in Health Care supplement, pp 8–15.

Hewison, A. (2003) "Leadership in health care", in *Management for Nurses and Health Care Professionals Theory into Practice.* Blackwell Science forthcoming, pp 127–128.

Lucas, E. (2000) "Tooling up for Leadership", *Professional Manager*, Institute of Management Vol. 9 Issue (6 September).

Mullins, L.J. (2002) *Management and Organisational Behaviour (Sixth Edition)*, Harlow, Prentice Hall.

National Assembly for Wales (2001) *Improving Health in Wales. A Plan for the NHS with its Partners.* Cardiff, TSO.

National Audit Office (2003) *Achieving Improvements Through Clinical Governance: A Progress Report on Implementation by NHS Trusts* www.nao.org.uk.

PDQ (2002) *Leadership in the West Midlands* Partnership for Developing Quality, NHSE West Midlands (June).

Scottish Executive (2000) *Our National Health: A Plan for Action, a Plan for Change.* Edinburgh, TSO.

Smith, J., Walshe, K. & Hunter, D. (2001) "The 'redisorganisation' of the NHS", *British Medical Journal*, Vol. 323 No. 1 (December) pp 1262–1263.

Tremblay, M. & Dunn, L. (2002) "Leading leadership: navigating the leader's journey", *National Nursing Leadership Programme Newsletter* (Autumn/Winter) NHS Leadership Centre, Department of Health London.

Werrett, J., Griffiths, M. & Clifford, C. (2002a) "A regional evaluation of the impact of the leading an Empowered Organisation Leadership Programme", *Nursing Times Research*, Vol. 7 No. 6 pp 459–470.

Werrett, J., Griffiths, M. & Clifford, C. (2002b) *Leading an Empowered Organisation Programme in the West Midlands: Evaluation Report*, School of Health Sciences, University of Birmingham.

West, M. (2002) "The HR factor", *Health Management*, Vol. 6, No. 6, pp 13–14.

Wilkin, D., Gillam, S. & Smith, K. (2001) "Tackling organisational change in the new NHS", *British Medical Journal*, Vol. 322, No. 16 (June) pp 1464–1465.

Wilson Barnett, J. (2003) "The achievement of more mature professional working relationships will benefit nurses' morale and enhance patients' well-being", *NT Research,* Vol. 7, No. 6, pp 471–472.

Woolnough, H. & Faugier, J. (2002) "An evaluative study assessing the impact of the leading an Empowered Organisation Programme" *Nursing Times Research*, Vol. 7, No. 6, pp 412–427.

CHAPTER ELEVEN

Opportunity knocks

Leadership development for allied health professionals and clinical scientists

John Edmonstone

In 2001 the then NHS Executive Trent Regional Office was busy extending the provision of the Leading an Empowered Organisation (LEO) programme from the nursing professions to cover Allied Health Professionals (AHPs) and Clinical Scientists – as foreshadowed in national policy on leadership development (DoH, 2000a,b). LEO is a three-day leadership development programme originally developed by Creative Healthcare Management in the United States, but later modified to the UK health context. It formed a major plank of the National Nursing Leadership Programme and has recently been evaluated positively (Woolnough & Faugier, 2002). LEO enables individuals to improve how they manage relationships and strengthens problem-solving and risk-taking skills. The experience of delivering LEO to nurses within the Trent Region suggested that the middle managers of LEO participants also needed investment in leadership development. It was also true that AHPs and Clinical Scientists historically had received very little access to leadership development opportunities at clinical, managerial or director levels. Finally, the creation of new health care organisations, such as Primary Care Trusts, and the merger of other organisations (typically into larger acute Trusts) all opened-up potential new career opportunities for AHPs and Clinical Scientists who were likely to be faced with key life and career decision-points and choices in relation to work/life balance.

In a fairly opportunistic manner, therefore, the Regional Office decided to supplement LEO provision with two other programmes, thus offering a "suite" of opportunities available to the professions concerned.

The new programmes

The two additional programmes commissioned were Leadership Effectiveness Analysis™ and Personal Directions™, based on diagnostic instruments developed by the Management Research Group (MRG) in the United States, but with a well-developed track-record of European norms.

Leadership Effectiveness Analysis (LEA) is a 360° diagnostic tool which provides participants with feedback on twenty-two leadership behaviours grouped into six functional work areas. Participants in the development programme were able to reflect upon their role, receive feedback and one-to-one coaching and develop an action plan that supported the development of their leadership effectiveness. LEA consists of a half-day briefing, a two-day development centre and a review day. Personal Directions (PD) is also a 360° diagnostic and provides a powerful assessment tool designed to help individuals explore carer development and personal growth issues. It provides individuals with rich feedback that helps them to explore their motivations, examine how these have affected the choices they have made in different areas of their lives and consider what actions they might take in future. PD can assist individuals to align their personal strengths with their job roles and responsibilities in order to increase their effectiveness and satisfaction. PD runs over three days and is also followed by a review day.

The programmes were commissioned by the Regional Office from the Centre for the Development of Healthcare Policy & Practice at the University of Leeds – which was then known as the Centre for Nursing Policy & Practice (CDNPP).

CDNPP had been commissioned by the Department of Health to deliver the LEO programme (through a regional infrastructure) to the nursing and AHP professional groups. It also had a number of years' experience of running LEA-based programmes and recent experience of designing and delivering PD programmes.

In order to help AHPs and Clinical Scientists make an informed choice from the suite of programmes two briefing days were held in October, 2001, at which those attending were able to hear presentations about LEA, PD and LEO and to ask questions with regard to the particular focus of the programmes in relation to themselves, their staff and their colleagues within their professions. A subsequent application process was managed by the Regional Office which involved:

- Completion of an application form which included details of the individual's sphere of responsibility and a case why the individual should attend the programme.
- Supporting authorisation from the applicant's line manager committing them to the release of the applicant for all programme dates.
- Screening of applicants against a set of agreed eligibility criteria.
- A random selection of those remaining.

Five LEA programmes were made available, with ten places on each. Three PD programmes were run, with six places on each. The programmes were run between December 2001 and June 2002.

Basic assumptions

Underlying LEA and PD are a number of basic assumptions regarding leadership and leadership development. They are:

- **Effective leadership can and should be present at all levels in the organisation.** It is not confined to people at the "top" of an organisation but permeates all areas and levels.
- **There is no single "one right way" to lead.** The diversity and complexity of people, organisations, challenges and opportunities are too great to allow for one approach which works in all situations.
- **Effective leadership is based on behaviour** – the ability to create organisational relationships which facilitate performance, co-operation, production and mutual job satisfaction.
- **Effective leadership behaviour is situational** – there are many roads to leadership effectiveness and the path taken will depend upon the demands of the specific situation the individual finds themselves in.

Programme design

The LEA programme began with a briefing day at which participants:

- Heard a full and complete description of the LEA diagnostic and the assumptions behind it.

- Completed the LEA questionnaire for themselves and identified the boss(es), direct reports and peers who would form the 360° element.
- Agreed a time-scale for returning the questionnaires to CDNPP, for transmission to Munich for analysis.

Some 6–8 weeks later the 2-day development centre was held. This event:

- explored the conceptual background.
- through use of a case study helped participants get used to the "language" of LEA.
- spelled-out what the LEA profile covered.
- provided 360° LEA feedback.
- provided one-to-one time for each participant with a CDNPP facilitator.
- encouraged participants to examine the role expectations of them by key others in the organisation.
- created helping pairs and trios for mutual support.
- encouraged the creation of personal action plans based on the 360° feedback and the opportunity for reflection which the development centre afforded.

The follow-up day, some four to six weeks later reviewed progress with action plans and reviewed opportunities for continuing leadership development.

The model for PD was slightly different, with no briefing day but a longer period of time for participants to be together in a more reflective mode, with time and space to explore feedback and ample one-to-one dialogue.

Evaluation

Owing to the limited "shelf-life" of the commissioning organisation (the Regional Office closed in March, 2003) and changes to the NHS architecture, with the emergence of Workforce Development Confederations and Strategic Health Authorities as major players in the leadership development field, a full-scale evaluation study was not possible. However, later in 2002 a small-scale evaluation study took place based on:

- Analysis of the evaluation forms which CDNPP routinely used following LEA and PD programmes. These seek data on such matters as programme, presentation, identification of useful aspects of the programme and identification of potential improvement areas.
- Focused interviews with all the CDNPP staff who delivered the programmes, concentrating on the situation prior to the events, the events themselves and then subsequent to the events.

Both programmes evaluated well, with LEA being considered as Very Good or Good by over 90% of participants in terms of programme, presentation, speaker and group interaction. PD achieved even better scores with 100% of participants regarding the programmes as Very Good or Good under these headings. The focused interviews produced some interesting and useful outcomes:

- There was probably an over-estimation of how much developmental activity participating professions had previously had access to. Moreover, the view of "leadership" by the AHPs and Clinical Scientists concerned seemed very much focused on their own professional group and the services which it delivered, rather than any "big picture" considerations of overall clinical and managerial leadership.

- For participants who had recently moved employer into PCTs, there was great difficulty in identifying both line managers and peers for the 360° analysis, in a new work environment which was experienced as very unstable. As a result, some participants put little weight on the perceptions of these (often new) immediate line managers.

- LEA and PD seemed to act as "triggers" for workplace dialogue on leadership issues, and this was recognised as useful and positive – if not always comfortable! The success of such dialogue seemed to turn upon two issues – the degree of skill of participants in presenting-back such data to bosses, peers and direct reports (and thus modelling helpful behaviour to them), and the reception from these groups. With regard to the latter, what was worrying was:

- Reported attitudes by a number of general managers that AHPs and Clinical Scientists were "not leaders" – simply deliverers of clinical services – a denial of the notion of clinical leadership and the equation of leadership with management only.
- When participants sought dialogue meetings with some line managers to discuss feedback results the latter became "elusive" – unable or unwilling to discuss such matters.
- When some meetings were set up some line managers either denied the validity of LEA and PD results or were reluctant to clarify specific behaviours.
- The model of leadership which emerged as being the norm in many workplaces was a narrow one, based on leadership being exclusively a management activity, and not a clinical one.

- Restructuring blight led to the preoccupation of many senior managers in setting-up new organisations and a high degree of anxiety with regard to their own role. This led in turn to a degree of cynicism on the part of such managers over programmes such as LEA and PD which were regarded by some as "navel-contemplation". Leadership and management were seen as *out there*, rather than as both *in here* and *out there* and the importance of self-reflection and understanding was denied.

- The increasing pace of work in employing organisations and the flatter structures which they had adopted meant that time and space for reflection had become, for many, a luxury, and was often not seen as "legitimate".

- There was little evidence of local employer support for programme participants. The notion of "organisation" seemed weak to these professionals who had experienced several restructurings and who had moved from one employer to another over short periods of time. It was unclear what support existed or how it might be accessed. There were some exceptions, and these seemed to be in organisations where:
  - There was an explicit local leadership strategy.
  - That strategy was consistent over a number of years.
  - The strategy worked "with the grain" of existing groups.
  - The strategy was resourced adequately.
  - A critical mass of people had similar developmental experiences.

Although some programme participants had agreed to meet again as Action Learning sets (in their own time) the majority felt that employers would need to give both permission and time for this to happen effectively. For these professionals, their occupational networks were more significant and enduring than their organisational ones – yet such networks were both fragmented and fragile, particularly in times of change.

• For the professions concerned there was a danger of a scarcity or victim mindset developing. The historical lack of access to developmental resources and activity had generated a culture of low (or no) expectations and the fragmented and fragile networks were not strong pressure-groups capable of turning this around. Nonetheless, some programme participants had grabbed the opportunity afforded them with both hands and were strongly pursuing their own leadership development.

Conclusion

The opportunities afforded to AHPs and Clinical Scientists in Trent were intended to support and enhance the mainstream leadership development opportunities which the LEO programme offered. While only a small number of individuals took advantage of the new programmes, the impact on these people was clearly a powerful one and the small-scale evaluation study has pointed-up many of the practical problems which both individual professionals and health care organisations face in enabling clinical leadership development.

References

Department of Health (2000a) *The NHS Plan: A Plan for Reform,* London, The Stationery Office.

Department of Health (2000b) *Meeting The Challenge: A Strategy for the Allied Health Professions,* London, The Stationery Office.

Woolnough, H. & Faugier, J. (2002) "An evaluative study assessing the impact of the leading an Empowered Organisation Programme", *NT Research,* Vol. 7, No. 6, pp 412–427.

CHAPTER TWELVE

Working with GPs and hospital consultants on developing clinical leadership in a health community

David Wilson and Helen Jones

This chapter describes work carried out to develop clinical leadership in health communities. It summarises why clinical leadership has become more prominent in the NHS in recent years; outlines the design of a programme involving GPs and hospital consultants working together on real issues; examines the impact of the programme, and identifies the lessons that can be drawn.

The clinical leadership context

In common with many other sectors, there has been a shifting emphasis from management to leadership in the NHS over the past decade, and more recently a particular emphasis on clinical leadership. This arises from the realisation that managers cannot deliver the fundamental re-design of the NHS that the Government has called for without effective engagement of clinicians. As Alan Milburn, the then Secretary of State for Health, put it at a conference in 2001:

> "The modernisation agenda for the NHS now makes clinical leadership imperative if the NHS Plan is to become effective. The simple truth is that the NHS works best when it harnesses the commitment and know-how of staff to improve care for patients ... what countless examples illustrate is that financial investment only works if it is matched by reform. And the essential ingredient that is needed is strong local leaders in charge of making that reform happen."

Changes in the design and delivery of health services pose several leadership challenges. (These challenges are not always successfully met, which explains much of the "patchiness" of NHS innovation.) Firstly, most innovation in health service delivery depends on leaders enlisting voluntary effort and collaboration from professional staff. A doctor's primary focus is individual patient care; a doctor doesn't lose his or her job for being uninterested in re-designing a hospital or department! Secondly, leadership of change requires knowledge of highly complex clinical processes – the operational knowledge to know what can be changed, and what will work in practice. Finally, most leadership of service change requires working in "multiple domains" (e.g. the worlds of patients, professions, managers, and politicians) and across both primary and secondary care – mainly without traditional managerial authority.

Clinical leaders such as general practitioners and hospital consultants are best positioned to meet these leadership challenges. They are more likely than "professional managers" to know the operation in-depth, and to have the expertise, credibility and respect that is required to build commitment to change. The question remains of how best to develop such clinical leadership.

The design brief for a clinical leadership development intervention

The work described below is from one health community, but draws on work which the authors have carried out in several other health communities over the past ten years.

Significantly, the design on which the intervention is based came from two NHS chief executives, David Fillingham (now chief executive of the NHS Modernisation Agency but formerly chief executive of Wirral Health Authority) and Frank Burns (chief executive of Wirral Hospital NHS Trust). They were looking for ways to develop the leadership skills of doctors. Alongside this requirement of developing skills for a group who had had almost no exposure to leadership and management training, they considered that there were two essential design requirements. Firstly, to do something for GPs and consultants *together*. Patient pathways need to operate smoothly between primary and secondary care, and many problems are at the "joins" between services. A joint programme would bring together doctors from the whole system and promote understanding and collaborative approaches to problems. Secondly, an intervention needed to deliver clear *service benefits* from any investment in training.

The world of leadership and management was an unfamiliar second language for most doctors and they had much scepticism about the value of management and leadership development – and even about management itself.

The overall objectives specified for the programmes therefore became:

- To develop the effectiveness of individual clinicians in leadership roles
- To improve understanding and partnership between primary and secondary care doctors
- To deliver service improvements.

The competencies clinical leaders require

The NHS gets steadily clearer on what it takes to be an effective clinical leader. The authors have carried out studies into clinical leadership competencies (for example, studies of Medical Directors in Scotland, and clinical leaders in Trent, and studies of GP leadership in primary care). Alongside this, substantial work has been invested in generic models, for example: the NHS national leadership qualities framework, a UK transformational leadership model (Beverley Alimo-Metcalfe), and the Leadership Effectiveness Analysis model (LEA)™ which is popular in several health organisations.

Our own studies enabled us to work with a simple but robust framework. Clinical leaders need:

- To understand what is going on (e.g. national policies that affect their service, the agendas of key stakeholders, and service developments and innovations)
- To see the way forward (whether in the sense of having a creative personal vision for a service, or vision in the sense of 20/20 vision – seeing how the story of policy change and modernisation is likely to unfold)
- To bring others with them, for example through using data, challenging questions and facilitation to prompt professional colleagues to look afresh at how processes work
- To turn plans and ideas into results, e.g. through effective change and project management, priority-setting and time management.

In addition to this linked leadership process, clinical leaders will be more effective if their general approach is one of developing and enabling individuals and teams. They will also need certain personal qualities, for example:

- Awareness of their personality and its impact on others
- The capacity to take the lead rather than simply react to events
- Emotional resilience and the capacity to stay calm in situations of conflict.

Finally, whilst not strictly being a competency, every study of what clinical leaders need mentions credibility in the eyes of colleagues – this coming from one's reputation as a clinician, one's integrity, and "gravitas" – or being taken seriously.

Key features of the design

It became clear to the authors that the most appropriate development method to use was Action Learning using group projects. Action Learning would enable doctors to learn about leadership through tackling real issues rather than through seeking to apply abstract concepts. In addition, the leadership challenges that GPs and consultants faced were what Reg Revans called "problems" rather than "puzzles". Puzzles have a neat single solution, whereas problems are characterised by imperfect data, multi-factor causes, different stakeholder perspectives, and difficult judgements. Problems are better approached through Action Learning than taught expert solutions.

It seemed that there would be more energy and learning if these real issues were tackled as group projects (in mixed groups of GPs and consultants) rather than individual projects. Group projects would enable individuals to learn together – through shared experience – in such areas as problem definition, team development, project management, and building support for change. Obviously it was important that groups selected projects that were both significant and feasible, and which they were highly committed to tackling.

As a further element of the design it made sense to support group work on projects with skills workshops in areas identified as important to clinical leadership roles.

Having two or three groups of around six participants would add energy and variety, and a degree of healthy competition between groups. (It was clear from early on that the desire to do something worthwhile for one's local health service was a very strong motivator).

The basic structure of the programme thus became:

- A two or three-day foundation workshop in leadership skills, plus time spent forming Action Learning groups, considering options for projects and identifying individual development priorities
- Six one-day meetings at approximately monthly intervals, each meeting combining a facilitated Action Learning meeting with a skills workshop to support group work. This time period enables action on projects to be developed and tested out, and learning to be properly embedded.
- A closing workshop of one or two days, to share outcomes and learning from projects with stakeholders, to agree project handovers and next steps, and to plan the continuing development of participants.

Certain principles were important to our design:

- Participants needed to be volunteers and to make a clear, informed choice that they wanted to participate. Accordingly, a pre-programme briefing meeting was held where people were invited to "taste the flavour of the programme" and to make a choice to opt in.
- Groups needed to choose their own projects rather than work on projects chosen by senior managers – however tempting this was. Group choice of projects was vital. Gaining the commitment of GPs and consultants requires that they work on some aspect of their local health service that they really want to change.
- Chief Executive involvement. Whilst selecting their preferred projects, it was vital that groups met regularly with the chief executives and other sponsors of the programme to make sure that their proposed projects were viable and worthwhile.

- Facilitators had to be responsive to the individual needs of the participants and to the issues which arose in the Action Learning groups – rather than offering a "package".

An example of an Action Learning project

The example is drawn from a recent programme designed on the structure and principles described above. The project chosen by the group of GPs and consultants was to examine medical emergency admissions at an Acute NHS Trust and particularly how these worked "out of hours".

The group initially pooled their knowledge to describe how the current admissions process worked. For example, if an elderly person had a fall at the weekend, a call would be made to a GP "out-of-hours" number, and an on-call GP would be driven to the patient's house. This journey might take an hour or more when the patient lived at the edge of the health district. It was likely that the GP did not know the patient, had no notes, and no access to testing facilities. A decision would therefore be made to admit to hospital and an ambulance would be called. The patient would be admitted to a ward where, typically, for a weekend admission, it would take a couple of days to get tests taken, and a diagnosis and treatment plan completed. At weekends, things were further slowed down by the unavailability of the Rapid Response Team, and, on a Sunday, ambulance transport. There could then be further delays due to waiting for an ambulance to be available to transport a patient home.

The topic was chosen because it was seen to be a waste of GPs' time, an inefficient and slow process, and poor for patient care, especially when patients were admitted to and kept in hospital unnecessarily. When the topic was tested out with the Chief Executives of the Acute Trust and Primary Care Trust (PCT), it was established that it was significant, and that clinical leaders were critical to its success. It was also seen as dovetailing with other work rather than duplicating it.

In defining the scope of the project, the group originally thought that a classic process mapping approach was essential. However this would take a long time, and was beyond the capacity of the group. Fortunately, a major emergency care mapping and re-design exercise had been launched by the Acute Trust. Action Learning group members attended one of the mapping workshops and were able to confirm and build on the group's initial diagnosis of how the process worked and its various gaps and bottlenecks.

There followed a phase of looking at innovation elsewhere and considering what literature to search and what data to collect. The project seemed a bit indeterminate, and group's energy and confidence started to dip. This phase was cut short by a proposal from one of the group, a Consultant Physician – who had a strong "Active Experimenter" learning style. He suggested that collecting data could go on for months, if not years. Perhaps the most useful and interesting thing the group could do was to test out a different process as a small-scale pilot within the sphere of responsibility of the consultants in the group. This would be on the lines of the Plan-Do-Study-Act (PDSA) cycle that is popular with GPs.

The proposal was to try out an alternative medical assessment process over a single weekend, and to evaluate the results. The process would give GPs in the out-of-hours service the option of referring a patient who had fallen to a Consultant Physician (via a mobile phone call) – rather than to the admissions ward. The Physician would be based in A&E, and would have the support required to give a rapid assessment and treatment plan – by way of test facilities, pharmacy, and home support. This would prevent unnecessary admissions to hospital.

This approach immediately appealed to the group. The Consultant Physician from the group proposed a pilot weekend when he was on-call, and GPs in the group transferred their shifts so that they could staff the out-of-hours service on the same weekend. Emphasis was placed on identifying and communicating with the wide range of stakeholders affected by the pilot. The support of the chief executives enabled the required resources to be negotiated, for example weekend availability of the Rapid Response Team. This work enabled the group to learn more about how the current process worked, for example contact with an Ambulance Manager revealed that it was not in fact necessary for GPs to visit the patient before ordering an Ambulance to bring them to hospital.

The weekend pilot was carried out, with only a small number of hiccups. For example, an out-of-district set of GPs had not been adequately informed and a supply of drugs had to be garnered because the Pharmacy requirement had been overlooked. The weekend was felt by group members to have been dramatically successful – in terms of patients being given a better, faster service and kept from an unnecessary hospital admission.

Results were evaluated, by means of identifying those patients who had not been admitted to hospital during the weekend, and following up these patients to check that outcomes were satisfactory.

Results were shared at a meeting of key stakeholders, and were very well-received. If the number of patients on the pilot weekend who were enabled to return home rather than being admitted was projected to a whole year, then the money involved amounted to millions of pounds. Notably, the Community Health Council representative said that the pilot offered a big improvement in the quality of patient care and pointed the way forward. The project provided local evidence that a different process was feasible and desirable, and produced advocates and champions for such a change in the consultant and GP group members.

Careful consideration was given to how to learn from and hand-over the project. For example, the issue of gaining commitment from other Physicians to new ways of working would be considerable. One of the group was appointed Clinical Director for Emergency Care shortly after the programme, enabling skills learned to be put into immediate use in a key position. The full-scale introduction of a new Medical Assessment process is planned for a year from now, as part of a wider emergency care modernisation programme

The group paid attention to what they had learned from tackling the project. For example – the need to understand how a process actually works, rather than to assume you know; that you can never pay too much attention to checking who the stakeholders are and communicating with them; that doing something small-scale and studying it creates more momentum than just collecting data; that it is much more productive to work on things that are high on the agenda of people like the chief executives; that a project goes through emotional peaks and troughs, and you have to keep going; and that GPs and consultants working together is a great engine for innovation in a local health service.

Evaluation

The programmes for the health community in the example above were evaluated through several means. Firstly, traditional reaction-level evaluation sheets gained participant views on the extent to which programmes met their three objectives. Responses were excellent. Secondly, the outcomes achieved from projects have been monitored. In most cases, project implementation has continued successfully, but in one momentum was lost. Thirdly, chief executives (the sponsors of the programmes) have judged their impact on clinical leadership in their health community. In respect of the Acute Trust, every Consultant who has been through a programme is currently in a specific clinical leadership role, part of a conscious strategy by the chief executive to build a "critical mass" of good clinical leaders . There is in-house support for continuing development of leadership skills. In respect of primary care, GPs typically said that their practices have been improved by attendance on the programme, but expressed dissatisfaction about how GPs were engaged in the Professional Executive Committee (PEC) of the PCT. This problem has now been addressed by creating a new clinical leadership role of "PEC Associate". PEC Associates will take on specific leadership responsibilities, e.g. for implementing a National Service Framework.

GP and consultant participants on the programmes recently took the initiative to call a conference with the chief executives and senior managers of the Acute Trust and PCT to discuss what helped and hindered effective clinical leadership in their health community. In collaboration with managers, they identified various improvement actions – having more cross-representation and joint policy meetings of the Hospital Clinical Board and the PEC; twinning PEC Associates and Clinical Directors to work as joint leads on specific modernisation programmes; and using the Action Learning/PDSA approach as a regular methodology for introducing change.

A further Action Learning programme is planned, and the approach is seen as an efficient and powerful way of developing a cadre of clinical leaders, working in partnership, and delivering real improvements on the ground. One of the chief reasons for the success of the programmes is something not so far mentioned – that working together on real issues in this close and informal way is enormous fun. People develop good friendships and this stands them in good stead for the future

Wider learning

The authors have run a dozen programmes using this design, in four different areas, with over 20 Action Learning groups of GPs and consultants.

Several things have been learned. Firstly, whilst many health communities want to run joint GP/consultant programmes, the level of collaboration between PCT and Acute Trust chief executives required to sponsor a joint programme is less common than one might assume. Secondly, for programmes to make a sustained difference, Action Learning groups projects must be "nested" in broader programmes of change, themselves nested within a strategic direction established by chief executives and Boards. Thirdly, one must not be too ambitious about what one can load onto these programmes. Attempts to specify the projects groups should work on or to add other professions, managers and social services to the basic mix of GPs and consultants – whilst appearing rational – have always weakened a programme.

The effective engagement of clinicians is still very near the top of the NHS agenda. As the introductory discussion indicated, effective clinical leadership at local level is vital to realising benefits from increased health investment. The joint GP/consultant Action Learning programme is an effective and powerful intervention for developing such leadership.

CHAPTER THIRTEEN

Succession planning at the University Hospital of North Staffordshire

Helen Green & Lesley Downes

Introduction

The University Hospital of North Staffordshire (UHNS) is a large 1,300-bedded acute NHS Trust based in Stoke-on-Trent. It serves a population of approximately half-a-million in North Staffordshire including the urban population of Stoke-on-Trent and the rural Staffordshire Moorlands area. The Trust is a regional centre for neuro-surgery, cardiac surgery, renal disease and neonatal and paediatric intensive are. The hospital presently is split over two main sites, which are within close walking distance of each other. However, a Private Finance Initiative (PFI) build over the next five years will bring all services together onto one site. This development, titled 'Fit for the Future' is more than just a new building – it incorporates a health economy approach to delivering the best health care possible for the population of North Staffordshire and requires leadership that can meet that vision.

The Trust employs approximately 2,200 nurses and midwives in its five divisions. Each division has a Professional Head of Nursing with the Women's and Children's Division also having a Professional Head of Midwifery. Although structures within the Divisions vary, it is not uncommon that the ward and departmental managers report directly to the Professional Head of Nursing for professional issues. These posts are, therefore, crucial to the maintenance of standards and the modernisation of nursing and midwifery to meet the demands of the present day NHS.

Investment by UHNS in the role of the Senior Clinical Nurse or Midwife (Modern Matrons) and the Consultant Nurse has proceeded over the last two years so that there are now 16 Senior Clinical Nurses or Midwives in post and three Consultant Nurses. Since these Senior Clinical Nurses and Midwives have been in post their roles as the focus for improvements in their 'patch' has become increasingly important. The Consultant Nurses help the organisation to look at new ways of working and to establish activities that can modernise nursing care and reduce junior doctors' hours. More Modern Matrons are to be recruited and there are plans for further Consultant Nurses and Midwives.

The nature of the problem

It was while considering recruitment to these senior nursing and midwifery posts that the senior nursing team, led by the Deputy Chief Executive/Chief Nurse, realised that there was not, at that time, a way that nurses and midwives within the organisation could easily gain the kind of experiences that would be required if they were to progress to more senior posts. The Trust had already invested heavily in leadership development courses for nurses and midwives which ensured that these practitioners were well-versed in the management of change and modernisation agendas within their own work environment. However, these courses did not enable the nurses and midwives to gain a more strategic view of the organisation which would be required by Professional Heads of Nursing or Midwifery in particular, but also the Senior Clinical Nurses and Midwives and in the Consultant Nurse and Midwife roles. Should a number of Professional Heads of Nursing or Midwifery leave the organisation at the same time would there be people within the organisation who could easily step into their shoes? The answer to that question was felt to be 'Not very likely'. Experience had also shown that for some senior nursing and midwifery roles there was not a plethora of external candidates. This was particularly the case with the Senior Clinical Nurse and Midwife posts, which were advertised at the same time that other NHS Trusts were trying to recruit to such posts. For some of these posts three separate attempts to recruit had been made. The value of 'new blood' within the organisation is recognised, but in the present climate obviously cannot be guaranteed.

A succession planning programme

The concept of a succession planning programme for nurses and midwives at UHNS was therefore considered to be an appropriate way forward. Succession planning is a more popular concept in the United States than the United Kingdom. There, best practice organisations use succession planning to develop and maintain strong leadership (Butler & Roch Tarry, 2002). Abrams (2002) suggests that senior management succession planning is a vital part of an organisation's strategic plan. It can be argued that succession planning is not only about filling future positions but should be seen in broader terms as being about developing people for future roles (Smeltzer, 2002). Succession planning is not about guaranteeing candidates posts, but about ensuring there is a pool of people eligible to apply for posts (Tyler, 2002). It is a proactive identification of leadership talent before the need for it arises (Bower, 2002). Certainly, these were the views of succession planning adopted by the senior nursing team at UHNS. The programme is about enabling the pool of management talent to be swelled without preparing candidates for specific posts or even guaranteeing them a promotion. It is made clear to all candidates that if the programme enabled them to 'think outside of the box' in order to do their present job more successfully then that was a positive outcome. However, it was also anticipated that there would be several people at the end of the programme who could be short-listed for senior positions. Smeltzer (2002) argues that in its broadest developmental context succession planning is not about making people think that you are lining them up for a particular job. It was also made clear that if people undertook the succession planning programme and then found a job in another organisation that this would also be regarded positively. However, there is evidence to suggest that the existence of succession planning programmes can encourage employees to stay with an organisation (Smith, 2002).

Identifying candidates for succession planning is not necessarily an easy task (Grab, 1996). Existing managers may be reluctant to put candidates forward whom they think would take their own job (Abrams, 2002; Greene, 1992), particularly if those candidates might do the job better than they do (Kaminsky, 1997). Although not always the favoured approach (McElwain, 1991) we asked existing managers in the form of the Professional Heads of Nursing and Midwifery to put forward those candidates that they felt had potential to be future leaders within the organisation. Eight candidates were put forward for the initial succession planning programme. However, one candidate later withdrew from the programme for personal reasons.

It was important that the senior management team showed their commitment to the succession planning process. If the senior team did not show such commitment then it was unlikely that the rest of the organisation would either (McElwain, 1991).

The importance given to the succession planning programme by the Deputy Chief Executive and the Associate Director of Nursing at UHNS was clearly apparent. They ensured that they were present at regular intervals during the succession planning formal education process, provided an external management consultant to facilitate some of the programmes and ensured that all the succession planning programme participants could spend time away from the organisation, to reflect on where they were and where they wanted to get to. Candidates underwent psychometric profiling so that they could discuss what were seen as their strengths and weaknesses with an occupational psychologist. All of the Professional Heads of Nursing and Midwifery were involved in the programme to a greater or lesser extent. Candidates were told that they had been identified for their potential to undertake senior roles within the organisation and that the senior nursing and midwifery managers at the Trust wanted to help them realise that potential.

The three important aspects of a succession planning programme are:

1. Visioning
2. Mentoring
3. Networking

(Tahan, 2002; Bower, 2000)

Visioning

The *visioning* aspect of the programme at UHNS was undertaken by allowing candidates the space to really understand themselves, their qualities and their aspirations. This was assisted by the use of psychometric profiling, leadership style instruments and encouragement to think about and undertake activities that candidates would either previously have thought were "not for them" or that they did not have time for within their everyday job.

The formal succession planning programme was carried out over a year. Tyler (2002) identifies one of the common mistakes of succession planning programmes as that of seeing the programme as an event rather than a process. If candidates were going to be given a chance to undertake 'blue sky' thinking then they needed to be able to go away and undertake experiences, reflect on those experiences and then move on to further ones. Because the programme was a developmental process, it was anticipated that the visioning would not stop just because the formal programme ended. It was envisaged that the programme would help candidates into new ways of thinking which they would take with them into any future roles that they might undertake. The benefits of the programme should be seen within the organisation after the end of the programme even if the candidates do not move from their present positions.

Mentoring

Another important part of the whole process is *mentoring*. The mentor can be the role model, guide, teacher, coach or confidant of the candidate (Bower, 2000). Pulcini (1997) argues that future successes in nursing are dependent on senior nurses' ability to mentor future leaders. Considerable time was spent deciding on how the mentorship within the UHNS succession planning programme should be undertaken. The value of having mentors from within the organisation or having mentors from outside was debated. In the end it was decided that the senior nursing team would be assigned as mentors, but that if candidates wanted to find external mentors they would be supported in doing so. The senior nursing team undertook an analysis of their own leadership styles so that this could be shared with the candidates who then had an element of choice as to who should act as their mentor. There were some restrictions. Most of the candidates were well known to their own Professional Head of Nursing or Midwifery who had indeed nominated them for the programme. It was felt important that candidates should be encouraged to see other parts of the organisation and experience other people's views. Candidates were, therefore discouraged from having their own Professional Head of Nursing or Midwifery as their mentor. Also, it was felt that, except in exceptional circumstances, mentors should not have more than one mentee. The enthusiasm for the programme by the senior Nursing and Midwifery team meant that there was never a need to have more than one mentee for each mentor.

The pattern of meetings between mentors and mentees was left to each pair to organise, with the onus being on the mentee to initiate meetings. It was expected that mentors would take the responsibility of their role seriously and ensure that they made time within their busy work schedules to meet with their mentee. Candidates had documentation to complete whilst on the programme and the mentors had to help them complete these. The paperwork mainly comprised a requirement for objective-setting and action planning with stage evaluations as to how well objectives were achieved and whether they still remained appropriate. The formal part of the reflective process was used to monitor progress. However, there was no requirement to keep notes of every meeting and the informal process of reflection and discussion was seen to be at least equally valuable to the candidates.

Networking

Networking opportunities were provided throughout the programme. Regular study days and workshops were provided throughout the year so that candidates could network with each other, something they saw as very important. Speakers from within the organisation were asked to come and discuss their role within the organisation and particularly what they did to fit in with the aims and objectives of the organisation and the Government's health agenda. Candidates were encouraged to shadow senior managers, to attend senior management meetings (which they may not have previously had access to) and to undertake what in the legal field is called 'second seating' (Woodhouse, 2002). This is where the candidate undertakes a role with a more experienced person at their side ready to take over should the need arise. Candidates asked for mentors and other managers to review their performance in activities such as chairing meetings, negotiating with seniors and so on, so they could get feedback on their own performance in areas where they were less experienced.

One of the problems of succession planning is seen as the tendency for existing leaders to mould potential successors in their own image

(Kaminsky, 1997). One way around this is to encourage exposure outside the organisation. The succession planning programme candidates went on visits to the Nursing and Midwifery Council and to a local bakery to look at how different organisations managed what they did. Individual candidates were also encouraged to arrange their own trips to any organisation they wished to visit with the Trust paying travel expenses and providing time as necessary.

Outcomes

Bower (2000) considers that the following questions should be asked to determine whether a succession planning process is working:

- Has a pool of talented persons who could fill openings in leadership been identified?
- Do these persons have the qualifications necessary to chart the future direction of the organisation, division, unit or department?
- Have the CEO, vice presidents or directors taken responsibility for mentoring the succession talent?
- Are the persons being mentored satisfied with the mentoring experience?
- Are the mentors satisfied with the protégés success?
- Have contingency plans been developed if mentored persons move onto other positions/places?
- Have the mentored persons who were hired been satisfactory?

Within the organisation it would appear that a pool of talented individuals with the appropriate qualifications has been identified. Two of the candidates on the succession planning programme are now Professional Heads of Nursing. These candidates had to go through the same selection process as other candidates, including external candidates. They had to be successful at an assessment centre and be interviewed in the same way as all of the other applicants. Other succession planning candidates have also changed their role since being part of the programme, which meant that more than half of them had a career change either before the end or soon after the succession planning programme ended.

The senior nursing and midwifery team, at the request of the Deputy Chief Executive, did prioritise the mentoring of succession planning candidates and at the evaluation of the programme this was one of the most positive things which was identified about the way the programme was organised. Whether the mentors are happy with the success of their protégés is still a little early to assess. Obviously, with the number of participants that have had career moves the programme could be said to be successful. However, only one programme has been completed and it is difficult to be sure that the programme was the reason for the candidates being successful in their aspired career changes and that these changes would not have happened anyway. For this reason, the Trust is working with the external consultant to identify methods of evaluating the impact of the programme on the organisation.

Mentees, as mentioned above, reported the relationship with their mentors as being one of the strongest parts of the programme. They reported that they had been able to discuss situations that had occurred while they were at work and sometimes saw them from a completely different perspective after they had reflected upon them with their mentor. Mentors reported that they had been very happy with the mentoring process when they evaluated it at the end of the first succession planning programme. Many said that they had seen differences, particularly in the confidence of their mentee.

Whether contingency plans were in place if the participant moved away from the organisation was not really an issue in relation to the succession planning programme at UHNS. Many of the US programmes discuss succession planning for a particular position within an organisation (Tyler, 2002; Butler & Roche-Tarry, 2002; Greene 1992). However, the programme at UHNS was not preparing individuals for specific roles but simply ensuring that nurses were developed so that both they and their managers felt that they were able to apply for more senior roles within the organisation. If the candidates then left the organisation this did not mean that there was a greater gap than if one of their colleagues who was not on the succession planning programme left the organisation.

Those who have taken up new positions have not yet been in them long enough to make any real objective assessment as to whether they are the appropriate people for the job. It would appear that the early signs are good. The long-term evaluation of the succession planning programme will be likely to produce more objective data in this respect. Overall however, using Bowers' (2000) criteria, the succession planning programme appears to have been worth the investment by the organisation. Certainly, it has been agreed that another group of candidates should be selected and commence the programme. Twelve nurses and midwives have embarked on a second succession planning programme, which uses the same format as previously with some minor amendments suggested by those who had completed the earlier one. This time psychometric tests will be completed at the beginning and end of the programme in order to see whether there are any significant changes over the course of the programme. The Trust is now in the process of organising a third cohort, which will be able to be accessed by Allied Health Professionals as well as nurses and midwives.

There are areas that could be strengthened within the succession planning process. These are mainly around the more objective selection of the candidates. Presently, Professional Heads of Nursing and Midwifery are asked for the names of those people who might benefit from the programme and who are in a position where they might next think of applying for a position in nursing and midwifery management. This requires the relevant people to be well known by the Professional Head. More work could be undertaken within the organisation to identify the competencies needed by the different senior management roles and matching candidates' competencies to these (McConnell, 1996). Only when there is some sort of a match would the candidate be accepted onto the programme. The organisation has gone some way to identify competencies against different roles, but there is still a way to go. The present competency of the individuals who might access the programme could also be more systematic. However, apart from this all the recognised attributes identified for the successful succession planning programme appear to be in place.

Conclusion

Girvin (1996) argues that the failure of nursing to produce leaders in sufficient quantities to meet the needs of Service is embedded in nursing's social and political history. Issues such as gender; the lack of value placed on leadership roles and the late awareness of the need for other than full-time work for women in their child-bearing years are all cited as influences that have had an effect on the lack of leadership development. Girvin argues that it was not until the almost complete removal of nursing from leadership positions at the time of the Griffiths reorganisation of the health service in the 1980's that the profession realised that nurse leaders would be missed. Recently, however, there has been a particular focus on leadership programmes at all levels of the NHS (DOH, 2000) and this includes the need for succession planning and career development. Rippon (2001) argues that a 'quick fix' on leadership is not possible and that time needs to be invested in preparation and good groundwork to set a healthy base for the future growth of leaders in the Health Service. Leadership development within the Trust is considered to be paramount for the provision of effective care for patients both now and in the future. The succession planning programme at the University Hospital of North Staffordshire is one of the ways used to nurture the leaders of the future and to try and ensure that when a senior post is ready to be advertised there is a pool of applicants who are able to apply. The programme has required investment both in terms of time and financial resources. However, it is anticipated that this will be returned with interest if future vacancies are quickly filled and if there is not to be a "rudderless ship" within departments on the departure of a manager because the organisation was not prepared.

References

Abrams, M. (2002) "Succeeding at succession planning", *Health Forum Journal,* Vol. 45, No. 1, pp 27–28.

Bower, F. (2000) "Succession planning: a strategy for taking charge", *Nursing Leadership Forum,* Vol. 4, No. 4, pp 110–114.

Butler, K. & Roche-Tarry, D. (2002) "Drawing a blueprint for succession", *Provider,* November, pp 51–53.

Department of Health (2000) *The NHS Plan: A Plan for Reform, A Plan for Success,* London, Department of Health.

Girvin, J. (1996) "Leadership and nursing: part three: traditional attitudes and socialisation", *Nursing Management,* Vol. 3, No. 3, pp 20–22.

Grab, W. (1996) "Succession planning: how to perpetuate your leadership", *Hospital Material Management Quarterly,* Vol. 18, No. 1, pp 61–65.

Green, J. (1992) "Hospitals struggle with the changing of the guard", *Modern Healthcare,* Vol. 22, No. 22, pp 20–22.

Kaminsky, R. (1997) "Succession planning: a long-overlooked need", *Caring,* Vol. 16, No. 4, pp 76–77.

McConnell, C. (1996) "Succeeding with succession planning", *The Health Care Supervisor,* Vol. 15, No. 2, pp 69–78.

McElwain, J. (1991) "Succession plans designed to manage change", *HR Magazine,* Vol. 36, No. 2, pp 67, 69, 71.

Pulcini, J. (1997) "Succession planning: from leaders to mentors: an open letter to experienced nurse practitioners' leaders", *Clinical Excellence for Nurse Practitioners,* Vol. 1, No. 6, pp 405.

Rippon, S. (2001) "Nurturing nurse leadership: how does your garden grow?", *Nursing Management,* Vol. 8, No. 7, pp 11–15.

Smith, E. (2002) "Leadership development: the heart of succession planning", *Seminars for Nurse Managers,* Vol. 10, No. 4, pp 234–239.

Smeltzer, C. (2002) "Succession planning", *Journal of Nursing Administration,* Vol. 32, No. 12, pp 615.

Tahan, H. (2002) "Relationship management: a key strategy for effective succession planning", *Seminars for Nurse Managers,* Vol. 10, No. 4, pp 254–264.

Tyler, L. (2002) "Succession planning: charting a course for the future", *Trustee,* Vol. 55, No. 6, pp 24–28.

Woodhouse, B. (2002) "Succession planning: lessons from the legal field", *Seminars for Nurse Managers,* Vol. 10, No. 4, pp 269–273.

CHAPTER FOURTEEN

Coaching clinical leaders for change

Sue Inglis & Jay Bevington

Introduction

Clinical leaders are increasingly at the forefront of changing practice and modernising services. Whilst traditional development programmes and training have tended to focus on management capability and leadership development, the 'Coaching for Complex Change Programme' (CCCP) programme designed by the Learning Alliance (a virtual service improvement team) focuses upon equipping clinical leaders with the skills, capability and understanding to manage complex change projects. The main aim of the CCCP is to deliver and spread sustainable change within health and social care communities.

Drawing from our experiences of working with many NHS organisations in the North of England, the Learning Alliance identified a significant gap in the development of clinicians. The changing nature of organisations, flatter hierarchies, new organisational concepts (shared services, lead commissioners etc) and a loss of tacit knowledge meant that traditional nurturing relationships had little opportunity to develop (Carter, 2001). In particular, there appeared to be a specific need for clinical leaders to have a greater understanding of how to work with the human dimensions of change – a skill area that was regarded as fundamental to the success of modernisation activities. In order to address this the 'Coaching for Complex Change Programme' was developed.

In this chapter we discuss the concept of coaching; its application within the CCCP programme and the experience of those who attended the Learning Alliance programme.

What is the 'Learning Alliance'?

The Learning Alliance is a virtual team, the focus of which is to support NHS and social care organisations in order to help them to modernise services and manage change effectively and thus to improve users' experience of those services.

The Learning Alliance has three core business processes:

- Training and development for service improvement
- Spread and sharing of good practice
- Bespoke OD intervention and support.

The Learning Alliance works through Strategic Health Authorities to ensure that capacity is directed at the most challenging agendas across a health and social care community. As part of the training portfolio the Coaching for Complex Change Programme is offered.

Why coaching?

"You see things as they were and say why – but I dream of things that never were and say why not?"

George Bernard Shaw

The term "coach" is from the French and means 'a vehicle to transport people from one place to another' (Goldsmith *et al.*, 2000). In the context of the NHS, coaching can be used to 'turn the things people do at work into learning situations, in a planned way under guidance' (Fleming & Taylor, 1999).

Coaching does not tend to be routinely available within the NHS and it is especially difficult for clinical leaders to access this kind of service improvement support. Many leadership development programmes within the NHS have focused on the 'sheep dip' approach, where a number of individuals are all exposed to the same basic information with the expectation they will synthesise this knowledge and that this will affect change for improvement. Executive coaching is slowly being used within the NHS (although currently mainly offered to senior personnel) and there is an evidence base from private sector organisations that coaching can change behaviour and improve performance (CMI/CFL, 2002).

The need to work intensively with clinical leaders and enable them to improve their personal effectiveness was a driver for the development of the CCCP.

The CCCP looked at developing individualised support for practitioners. The lack of availability generally for this sort of programme may be due to the time-intensive nature of the approach and the need to commit to work with individuals over time. Many people consider coaching to be a face-to-face activity, contracted between two people. The basis for the CCCP is that we all learn from each other and we can therefore increase everyone's understanding by accepting we all teach and we all learn. Therefore the participants were as much coaches as the facilitators. This shifted the emphasis from an expert consultancy perspective towards mutuality of learning. Through expert facilitation the group were able to share expertise, knowledge and practical experience of managing change. This accelerated their learning through exposing them to theoretical knowledge that underpinned their practical 'know how' and providing an environment of questioning and challenge. Inviting a multi-organisational group of individuals all working in the sphere of service improvement enabled differing organisational approaches to be compared and contrasted. We used Action Learning techniques to draw out and question the assumptions attendees made about their own project, organisation and self (Pedler, 2001).

Programme overview

The programme is available to middle managers, executives, clinicians and a broad range of professionals who are responsible for implementing complex service improvement projects within health and social care communities based in the north of England. The ultimate aim of the CCCP is to 'spread sustainable change' within health and social care communities. The programme seeks to support the delivery of the modernisation agenda by enabling change leaders to:

1. Have access to high quality change management and organisation development expertise that is both evidence-based, practically-focused and tailored to the specific needs of each delegate attending the programme.

2. Reflect upon the challenges they are experiencing within their organisations and design a strategy to successfully resolve these difficulties, with the aim of achieving sustainable behavioural change and real cultural change.

3. Work towards becoming effective and high-calibre change agents, thereby increasing the capacity and capability for sustainable change within their respective organisations.

CCCP is a consultancy-based programme, delivered over a period of approximately 4 months. Delegates are required to attend three workshops over this time and to undertake work on their change projects in the interim with the support of the Learning Alliance. The content of each workshop is bespoke to allow the diverse needs of each group to be addressed effectively. Each programme is restricted to a maximum of 6 people to ensure that participants are given sufficient time to fully explore their particular change project and the models and techniques being discussed. Two coaches support each cohort.

Once a place is allocated, the attendee is sent pre-work to complete. This work relates to their project, issues and an outline of what they hope to achieve from attending the programme. This information is used to inform the coaches' preparation around possible subject areas that may wish to be addressed or worked through. The session is run using Action Learning principles with the coaches acting as facilitators.

A review of learning needs at the end of each session enables the coaches to undertake preparation on specific subjects identified by the group for the following sessions, these forming part of a seminar programme. The group also have access to the coaches between the programme days, for telephone support or face-to-face coaching. The attendees also act as advisors and support for each other, forming their own small network. This is actively supported by the Learning Alliance. The coaches act as a conduit for information between participants as well as posting interesting articles, papers or references that may be of use to the group.

Evaluation

The programme has been run for two years and at the end of 2002 an evaluation was undertaken by the Learning Alliance and the Centre for Business Excellence, University of Northumbria. Specifically, the evaluation process focused upon three key issues. The results of the evaluation are presented here:

1. What benefits did people get from attending the CCCP (impact analysis)?
2. What do people perceive the CCCP's critical success factors to be?
3. How could the programme be improved?

This evaluation shows the main findings from each of these three areas and makes several recommendations based upon participant feedback.

Methodology

A survey of 13 people who had attended a CCCP between April 2001 and April 2002 was undertaken. These 13 people were picked randomly from a total sample of approximately 25 participants. The evaluation was confined to those programmes that had been advertised as part of the Learning Alliance's Programme of Events. The longitudinal analysis consisted of a semi-structured interview, the content of which was based on a questionnaire devised by the Learning Alliance and the Centre for Business Excellence (see Appendix). The survey utilised both quantitative (Likert Scale) and qualitative methods (open-ended questions). In addition to the interview, informal comments and suggestions that had been made to Jay Bevington by different participants over the previous 12 months were integrated into the evaluation.

Benefits of the programme

The majority of people interviewed agreed that the CCCP had helped them to effectively address the specific change problem(s) that they had brought to the programme. Specifically, 7 and 8 people agreed that the programme had challenged them to reappraise the way they do things at work/gave them new insights and had enabled them to learn from others

Table 14.1: Level of participant agreement on a series of statements relating to cognitive and behavioural change reported several months after attending a CCCP

The CCCP has...	Strongly disagree	Disagree	Uncertain	Agree	Strongly agree
Helped me to effectively address the change problem(s) that I brought to the programme.				8	5
Challenged me to reappraise my way of doing things at work/gave me new insights.			1	7	5
Helped me to make changes in my workplace			1	7	5
Been valuable because it enabled me to learn from others and share experiences			1	8	4

and share their experiences respectively. There was variation on all the responses in a positive direction, with some attendees strongly agreeing that the CCCP had helped them to make cognitive and behavioural changes in their work (see Table 14.1).

As part of the qualitative analysis, various quotes from participants were recorded. Here are just a few:

> "Before attending the programme I was really stressed and didn't feel I could justify the time to attend the workshops but I'm really glad I did – it is one of the best things that has happened to me during my career in the NHS. Overall, the programme has really changed me. I've stopped trying to change everything today. I'm much better equipped to deal with things – I've gained new perspectives and can now see what is needed. I couldn't attend anything like this if I had to pay. It is brilliant that this sort of thing is being made available through the Learning Alliance."
>
> > Senior Nurse in the process of setting-up a new service in her Accident & Emergency Department at the time of attending the Programme

> "I have been involved in establishing a learning site which, at the time of the programme, involved 3 key people: myself; an IT manager; and

a clinician. Coaching For Complex Change made me realise that we hadn't mapped-out what we wanted to achieve at the beginning of the project. I took this back to the project team and consequently we've shifted from a team of enthusiasts to a high-level strategic partnership. We're now focusing on the whole health community, not just our PCT. Essentially, the programme shifted my thinking, acted as a trigger and made me realise the need to be more strategic."

Primary Care Senior Manager

"I have realised that I have gained more from the Programme than what I first thought and therefore the time invested has been really worthwhile. My colleagues and I thoroughly enjoyed all the workshops and got an awful lot from them. Since attending the course we have actively promoted much more ownership of the collaborative at a local level, which has been hugely beneficial. We also believe that there is some serious value in the framework that was used and consequently are beginning to use it as part of our own management structure."

Programme Manager from
one of the national collaborative programmes

"By enabling me to understand more about the nature of change, Coaching for Complex Change made me more reflective in my practice; more facilitative in style, and more confident of my own ability. Also, the course was instrumental in making me change my career path!"

General Manager of an Acute Trust

"The programme provides an environment free from risk so you can explore new ways of working. It is an excellent way of getting up to speed with the latest thinking on change management and related subjects."

Divisional Manager of a large Acute Trust

"Whilst I've always been good at getting other people to think "out of the box", this programme has helped me to do some "out of the box" thinking myself. I enjoyed being challenged, but never felt threatened, which is important. I would definitely recommend the programme because it makes you think about your own capabilities and leadership skills. I really got a lot from the whole experience."

Senior Quality Audit Co-ordinator

"Coaching for Complex Change enables you to see the 'wood and the trees!' I found the insights and stories from different sectors and industries introduced by the facilitators both invaluable and refreshing. I'm using the concepts and tools in my own Trust's Management Development Programme and have received lots of positive feedback already."

Human Resources and Development Co-ordinator

"One of the huge benefits I got from attending the course was that it gives you the opportunity to pick up lots of practical hints and tips from other members of the group. For example, I am dealing with 26 departments and experience difficulty in keeping up-to-date with everyone, asking them to complete formal reports, etc which they rarely do. A member of the group suggested I give out a one-page pro-forma at every meeting that has to be completed before people leave the room. This simple change works really well and has saved me plenty of time chasing people up. I've made some useful contacts, in particular a lady who has worked previously on the same thing I am now doing, so she has given me a lot of useful advice."

Booked Admissions Project Manager

"The programme helped me to understand a series of major changes in my working life better and enabled me to gain some sense of control and mastery."

Regional Head of Speciality

Critical success factors

Interviewees highlighted the following list of critical success factors (not presented in any particular order):

- The *small group format* enabled people to receive bespoke help in relation to their particular change project.
- The structure of the programme allowed participants to exclusively focus upon *one particular challenge* over a *reasonable period of time.*
- Access to the *latest techniques and models* from the literature on change management and associated disciplines, and the effective *translation of this thinking into practice.*

- Provision of a *secure, confidential forum* for debate and problem-solving.
- The use of Action Learning methodology.
- Skills of the facilitators – use of a *'process consultation' style* as opposed to simply giving generic advice and/or being too directive.
- Opportunity to *share experiences* with others and learn from the members of the group.
- Having access to a helpful resource *between workshops*.
- Learn about *different sectors* and industries.
- The provision of *high-quality venues* that facilitate the process of learning.

Continuous improvement

The Learning Alliance considers that evaluation is the cornerstone of quality improvement and commissioned the evaluation specifically to understand what changes needed to be made to improve the programme. Various critical themes emerged from the survey data. These are discussed below in descending order of priority. We have also included the actions that we agreed to take to address these issues to highlight the importance of committed action planning as part of an improvement cycle (see Table 14.2).

In addition to the above recommendations, it was also proposed that a CCCP Alumini Network be established from September 2002. This would have three key purposes:

1. Continued networking of previous programme participants.
2. Continued dissemination of the latest change management tools and techniques using an email platform.
3. A database of people who can act as change agents/advisers for staff approaching the Learning Alliance for help with similar issues.

The development of the Alumni Network has been arrested due to organisational changes within the NHS, specifically the demise of the former Regional Offices and Directorate of Health & Social Care. The Learning Alliance, in keeping with its core principle of capacity development, has forged ahead and developed a community of practitioners who

Table 14.2

Description	Comment(s)/recommendation(s)	Done
Group composition		
6 out of 13 people stated that the group dynamics, and consequently, the selection of participants was very important. Whilst some found the heterogeneous nature of the group (i.e. diverse professional backgrounds facing very different challenges) extremely valuable, others thought it was important for everyone within the group to have similar levels of seniority, leadership and change management experience and facing similar challenges.	With regard to the CCCP, 3 levels of group homogeneity can be identified: 1. CCCP run with people from the same organisation; 2. Group members chosen on the basis that they are all facing the same challenge; 3. Participants selected on the basis that they all operate at similar levels of seniority and experience. Option 1 is not favoured on the grounds that people attending from the same organisation are all governed by the same cultural variables. However, two CCCPs have been run on this basis and both were deemed to be successful by attendees. There might be a lot of potential in Option 2. CCCP could be used in contexts where people are facing the same issues. This model has already been used effectively with one collaborative programme and is about to be used with another. It would be difficult and time-consuming to undertake the screening process required in Option 3. However, it could be emphasised within the marketing literature that CCCP is an advanced-level programme requiring previous experience of managing change. Less-experienced people would be better-placed attending the introductory change management workshop featured on the Learning Alliance's Programme of Events. Realistically, Options 1 and 2 often co-exist, therefore, targeting one option will concurrently promote the other option.	✓

(continued)

Table 14.2 (continued)

Description	Comment(s)/recommendation(s)	Done
Duration of the programme		
5 out of 13 people interviewed commented that they found the programme to be too short. They indicated that it would be beneficial to have a follow-up day, approximately 3 months after the 3rd workshop. It was felt that this would further increase the sustainability of the changes they had introduced and promote further networking.	Introducing a fourth workshop to the programme could be considered but only post April 2003 when the next series of programmes are being planned and budgeted.	
Unstructured nature of the programme		
4 people found the workshops to be too unstructured and consequently did not know what to expect from attending the programme. They also felt that the lack of structure led to too many topics being covered which made it difficult to understand how the various parts of the programme fitted together.	The unstructured nature of the CCCP is intentional. The challenges that people present at the start of the programme are complex, dynamic and diverse, therefore, it would be inappropriate to standardise all the inputs. However, the CCCP could seek to cover specific themes. The themes that are deemed to add most value to NHS staff managing complex change projects at the current time are: • Effective management of the human dimensions of change (e.g. managing conflict, overcoming resistance to change, etc…). • Best practice in sustaining and spreading organisational change. • Models and techniques for achieving culture change. • Strategic concepts and tools (e.g. complexity science and polarity management). These themes are beginning to be integrated into the marketing literature. In addition, a letter will be sent out to all participants prior to the start of each CCCP detailing the aims of the programme; key themes and an idea of the contribution that each participant will be expected to make.	✓

(continued)

Table 14.2 (continued)

Description	Comment(s)/recommendation(s)	Done
Length of time between workshops		
Three people stated that the time between sessions (ie. 4 weeks) was too short to allow any meaningful progress to be achieved.	The length of time between each workshop has now been increased to 6 weeks.	✓
Size of the group		
Three people thought that the size of the group was too large.	This issue was raised by 3 members of a group of 8 people. All programmes have subsequently been restricted to 6 participants.	✓
Contact between workshops		
Two people commented that although it was stated at the onset that the facilitators would contact participants between sessions to offer their help and support, this did not always happen.	It can obviously be difficult contacting people due to the hectic schedules of programme participants and the facilitators. However, informal contact between sessions adds to the value that group members gain from the CCCP and should therefore be undertaken.	✓

have an interest and expertise in managing change. A number of shared learning events are held each year to discuss specific tools, techniques, strategic objectives and new learning that may be useful for practitioners working within the change agenda. The community of practitioners are bonded through a common interest in effective change management, especially developing productive human relationships to facilitate a changing culture.

Conclusion

The CCCP is a successful and effective product offered by the Learning Alliance, demonstrating significant impact over time. However, there is always room for improvement. Various recommendations outlined by the evaluation study have already been introduced and further improvements made. The strength of the programme appears to lie in the balance between providing timely theoretically-based skills development and coaching participants to implement these skills within the projects for which they are responsible.

The interactive nature of the programme; the development of capability and competence and the input of one-to-one coaching suggest a model of organisational development that has the potential to demonstrate real impact. Caution, based on the small sample is necessary, but anecdotal evidence and continued interest in the programme indicate that this approach is valued by participants.

Historically, the NHS has invested in leadership programmes with little evidence of organisational impact. Our experience of the CCCP suggests that individuals and organisations benefit more from bespoke individualised access to coaching and skills development. Coaching may appear to be labour-intensive. However the noticeable development of confidence; sharing of knowledge and learning and the application of new skills, makes a major impact on organisational competence and provides the opportunity for individuals to develop coaching skills thereby supporting others within an organisation mandated to deliver the modernisation agenda.

References

Carter, A. (2002) *Executive Coaching: Inspiring Performance at Work*. Institute for Employment Studies. Eastbourne, Anthony Rowe.

Goldsmith, M., Lyons, L. & Freas, A. (eds) (2000) *Coaching for Leadership: How the World's Greatest Coaches Help Leaders Learn*, San Francisco, Jossey-Bass.

Chartered Management Institute/Campaign For Learning, (2002) *Coaching at Work Survey*, London, Lloyds TSB.

Pedler, M. (2001) *Action Learning for Managers*, London, Lemos & Crane.

Fleming, I. & Turner, A. (1999) *The Coaching Pocketbook*. Hants, Alresford Press.

Appendix 1: Coaching for Complex Change programme delegate survey

Please take a few minutes to complete the following questions:

	Strongly disagree 1	Disagree 2	Uncertain 3	Agree 4	Strongly agree 5
The Coaching for Complex Change programme has… (Please tick the box that best describes you)					
1 Helped me to address the change problem(s) that I brought to the programme	❏	❏	❏	❏	❏
2 Challenged me to reappraise my way of doing things at work/gave me new insights	❏	❏	❏	❏	❏
3 Given me new confidence to approach things differently at work	❏	❏	❏	❏	❏
4 Helped me to make changes in my workplace	❏	❏	❏	❏	❏
5 Been a good use of my time	❏	❏	❏	❏	❏
6 Confirmed a lot of things that I already knew	❏	❏	❏	❏	❏
7 Met my expectations	❏	❏	❏	❏	❏
8 Been valuable because it enabled me to network with others	❏	❏	❏	❏	❏
9 Been valuable because it enabled me to learn from others and share experiences.	❏	❏	❏	❏	❏
10 Been disappointing.	❏	❏	❏	❏	❏

11 If you have made changes to your working life as a result of the CCC programme, please describe what these changes have been:

12 If you have not made any changes to your working life as a result of the CCC programme, please explain why this might be:

13 Please complete the following sentence:
    If I was running the CCC programme, I would…

14 Please indicate why you would or would not recommend the programme to others.

15 Are there any further comments/suggestions you would like to offer with regard to the
   Coaching for Complex Change Programme?

Thank you for completing this questionnaire.

CHAPTER FIFTEEN

Leading a vision for change in Northumberland: a case study

Ann Foreman, Karen Picking, Wendy Cowie, Sophia Martin and Nick Nicholson

Introduction

In 2000, the Chief Executives of all the Health and Social Care organisations in Northumberland identified a shared vision for change. This would involve strategic transformational changes across the whole health and social community. In order to achieve this, they identified the need to develop leadership capacity within all the partner organisations. An innovative leadership development programme for the whole health and social care system in Northumberland (but provided through Northumbria Healthcare NHS Trust) was launched.

By August 2003, Northumberland had developed a visionary strategy for health and social care. Major transformations of services across the whole system of care will create a modern and efficient service focused around patients, their pathways of care and the care-streams that support this care. The Northumbria Healthcare NHS Trust is a lead acute Trust and Northumberland Care Trust is one of the first two Care Trusts established in England for integrated Health and Social Care within four primary care localities. Both organisations reflect innovative and collaborative leadership across the whole system. The 200 clinical and professional leaders who have participated in the leadership development programme have significantly led this vision for change.

This chapter describes that vision for change in Northumberland and the need for collaborative transformational leadership to achieve this vision. It outlines the leadership development programme run by Northumbria Healthcare NHS Trust between 2000 and 2003 that supports this vision for change. It describes the programme and the innovative and creative approaches which provide a stimulating, challenging and supportive learning environment for transformational experiences in leadership development for participants. It includes both quantitative and qualitative evaluation of the programme.

The authors who have designed and facilitated the programme share what they have learned and outline plans to share, spread and sustain leading visions for change in this and other health and social care communities.

Leading a vision for change

Northumbria Healthcare NHS Trust is an acute Trust serving a large geographical area from North Tyneside, north to Berwick on the Scottish Border and west to Haltwhistle. Its population is around 500,000. Spanning the same geographical area, the Northumberland Care Trust was created in 2002 and incorporated the four earlier local Primary Care Groups (PCGs) and community care staff from Northumberland County Council Social Services Department.

Chief Executives from these local health and social care organisations were partners in building a shared vision of service development from 2000. This vision underpinned a partnership in strategic thinking and created an essential commitment that a new and multi-agency leadership development initiative should be established.

The purpose of the leadership development programme was to contribute to modernisation and change, and it was based on the recognition of a need to develop leadership capacity in *all* the partner organisations. The Chief Executives' vision created an agenda of closer union in delivery and management of services and of more collaborative working across the spectrum of health and social care settings.

The programme: a design based on good practice in leadership development

The intention of the programme design is to give participants an opportunity to analyse the realities of their own workplace as the basis for defining their personal leadership and change agenda; to introduce useful theory and generic leadership ideas, while offering inspiration to both

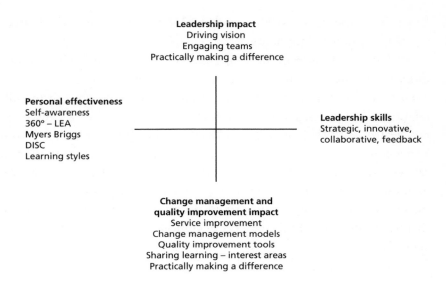

Figure 15.1: Programme design principles

innovation and creative thinking. A key element is to make the links back to the workplace through participant action and learning.

The delivery of the programme is based around four key features (see Figure 15.1). The Northumberland programme does not follow a set curriculum, but instead offers flexibility in order to meet individual and peer group needs, and to leave "design space" for self-management by the participants. Following a first diagnostic event, needs and priorities for development are identified in the form of a learning contract and the design of subsequent meetings is based upon these themes.

360° feedback

The developmental theme was emphasised from the outset by the use of a 360° feedback instrument, the Leadership Effectiveness Analysis (LEA)™ by all participants. As well as providing individual assessments of leadership skills and style, this instrument has also been used in a composite format, the Strategic Direction Questionnaire (SDQ), to research the key leadership behaviours required by our organisations (MRG, 2000). This is supplemented by other diagnostic tools such as the Myers

Briggs Type Indicator (MBTI)) and the DISC Personal Profile Analysis created by Thomas International.

All Northumbria leadership programmes are multi-disciplinary. Two different versions have been developed. The *Whole Systems* programme is open to leaders and potential leaders from all the professions in the different health and social care agencies (social services, primary care, mental health, and health commissioners) who learn together about leadership and also about issues in the management and organisation of services across the local health economy. A *Trust* version of the programme is run in parallel, enabling clinical leaders (clinical directors, nurses, heads of service, general and operational managers) to develop their leadership skills in the context of clinical service development in the acute Trust.

> "Nothing in my career development so far has given me the chance to learn in this sort of way – being alongside other disciplines, people from other organisations – and to listen and learn from them. They question things you haven't even thought of – and they can help you to see things you couldn't have worked out on your own."

> "You understand people better, and their part of the system, the issues and needs they have – and that is the start of working out how to co-operate and consult."

> (All quotes from senior leaders who participated in the programmes during 2002 captured by independent evaluation (Martin, S. (2003) Evaluation of Leading a Vision for Change Development Programme))

Twenty participants are recruited to each cohort of the programme. To earn nomination, participants must be in a leadership role within their own organisation, and have sponsorship of their Chief Executive or another senior Director. Participants need to have links with other senior colleagues, and there is a requirement that their workplace provides challenges and significant opportunities for change in leadership practice to be implemented, for the benefit of a team or network of other service development colleagues.

Strategic Direction Questionnaire (SDQ)

The SDQ instrument revealed a need to develop better strategic thinking capacity in the partner organisations in Northumberland, as well as developing peoples' innovation skills and making them less traditional in how they envision the future. The need for skills in communicating with energy and enthusiasm was also emphasised as key to building teams and creating followership. Analysis of participants' LEA™ reports showed both health and social care professionals with strong team skills, but whose leadership style depended on direct control and a strong managerial focus. Greater involvement, with a high emphasis on feedback and more co-operative approaches were called for in leading changes in service delivery; in finding a shared patient-focus, and in creating new organisation structures.

These needs represented significant development challenges for both the individuals and organisations concerned. These had to be addressed through designing a flexible and challenging programme which had top management support. This high-level sponsorship of leadership development was very significant, both in gaining resources to run the programmes, but also in creating a culture which gave "permission" for change in managerial styles and roles as people developed as leaders and moved outside more traditional professional and organisational boundaries and service domains.

> "I'm cynical about everything, but not about this. It increased my energy, it is liberating to get that sort of affirmation, and such good support, it is a challenge, but always such a constructive one."

Change management and quality improvement tools and techniques

Methodologies for change management, such as the European Foundation for Quality Management (EFQM) Excellence Model (Stahr *et al.*, 2000) and strategic thinking models and approaches; the ethics of leadership; patient-focused leadership; communication and interpersonal skills have all featured on learning set days. The Excellence model, in particular, provides an organisational framework against which organisations can assess and improve the quality of their services. Emphasis was placed upon the skills of personal development; building awareness of personal leadership styles; encouraging creativity and experiment through Action Learning. Throughout the programmes participants had contact with excellent speakers and practitioners with national and international profiles as leaders and teachers, but were also supported by a dedicated facilitator and coaching team which has provided an important continuity to the programme.

> "We heard about the new NHS plan, the new structure, all in the midst of the changes happening; it was an intensive seminar, a crash course in what was going to happen. And you were working on it alongside the managers affected, so you could appreciate the personal effect and upheaval it meant for them."

> "You were with a network of people from your new peer group – you could focus on working out how to do things, how to make things happen, interpret the new environment and the new ideas that were flying all over the place."

The participants were introduced to a raft of tools and techniques for change management and quality improvement. (see Table 15.1) Leaders on the programme were encouraged to explore and experiment in using these tools and then supported in this process through coaching. Each tool or technique will have potentially a different impact upon individual participants and they adopt them with differing degrees of interest and confidence.

The approach was further refined in the light of evidence provided for the NHS Leadership Centre by Paul Plsek, a major contributor to the

Table 15.1: Service Improvement Techniques

• EFQM	• Work and patient flow
• Polarity management	• Process mapping/pathways
• Demand and capacity	• Rapid learning cycles
• Simple rules/complex adaptive systems	• Process control charts/variation mapping
• Accelerated quality improvement	
• Pursuing perfection	• Care stream design
• Eliminate waste	• Theory of constraints
• Scenario planning/what ifs	• Change management theories

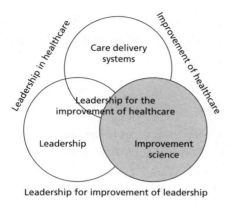

Source: Paul Plsek, Framework for the Leading Modernisation Programme

Figure 15.2: Framework for the Leading Modernisation Programme

Northumberland programmes over the three-year period. (Plsek, 2003) – see Figure 15.2.

Action Learning and coaching

Participants were supported in applying their learning through small Action Learning sets, many of which continued on as self-directed and self-managed, long after the formal programme was completed. They were also supported with one-to-one coaching.

> "Action Learning was very significant. You take real work issues into a learning set. There, you had to listen and ask questions. You sorted yourself out through that process of opening up, questioning, and being challenged by other people. You get ideas you'd never have even thought of."

Experiential learning and innovative learning methods

A variety of learning methods were offered throughout the programme. Creativity was encouraged through the use of large art boards and music. Experiential opportunities were positively received, examples being the Westminster Experience and the Transformation of the Royal Opera House for Excellence in Performance. Many participants regarded personal leadership journeys and private reflection explored on the wild beaches and moorlands of Northumberland as a particularly powerful and formative experience.

Participant stories

The programme's significance as an (often intense) personal development journey was evident. In most cases there was some variation on the theme of enhanced self-awareness and a focus on personal influence and style. There was also reference to learning being "whole-life" focused, and that it had been helpful to re-think such issues as career options. In the great majority of cases, however, the insights achieved are strongly evidential of a re-commitment by participants to the immediate demands of the workplace; to new and existing teams, and to the wider health and social care service of which they were a part.

Evaluation

Evaluation of the programmes is ongoing through rapid learning cycles of expert planning, trial and pilot, review and implement with action. Thus the programmes are continuously adapting. The programme was independently evaluated in 2002 (Martin, 2003). This study, based upon structured interviews, examined the impact of the programme on the participants, their teams and the organisation.

A leadership learning community with neighbouring Tees and North East Yorkshire NHS Trust (who have been providing both similar and additional new programmes) shares learning and resources across the two leadership communities. The underpinning of the Tees and North East Yorkshire programmes is:

> "to provide an opportunity for leaders and potential leaders to work with other professionals on their leadership skills, and issues, which have a significant impact on the delivery and organisation of Mental Health and Learning Disability services.

All of our programmes provide participants with time and space to reflect upon individual and potential team working across professional and organisational boundaries.

All of our development is based upon the following assumptions.

- Any training and development has as its main purpose to benefit patients and carers because that is what the NHS exists for (Jarrold, 1998)
- Experiential learning (Kolb, 1984) plays a major role in the development of individuals and groups
- The use of 360° appraisal and feedback is beneficial to leadership development (Alimo-Metcalfe 1998, Antomiani 1996)
- Access to mentoring and coaching ensures sustainable change to leadership behaviour (Sadler 1999)"

(Cowie, W. 2003)

All programmes, both in Northumbria and Tees and North Yorkshire are dynamic and interactive in nature, with the participants as key partners in shaping their learning. No two programmes are ever the same. Evaluation is based upon the framework as shown in Figure 15.3. The

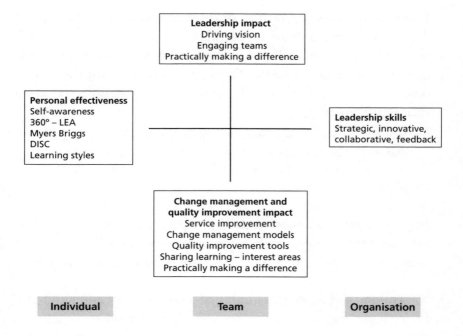

Figure 15.3: Evaluation framework

impact of the programme for each of the four aspects is considered at the three levels : individual. team and organisation.

Outcomes – leaders with new skills and attitudes

The regular evaluations have provided clear evidence of very high satisfaction with the learning process, the inspiration of speakers, and support of facilitators. The material covered was very largely judged to be relevant and practicable, with 90% of participants finding ideas and methodologies they could translate into their own workplaces and leadership practice. Throughout the programmes, there has been strong evidence of significant personal learning about leadership ideas being carried through into workplace behaviour.

Independent evaluation of the longer-term organisation outcomes, researched through work with past participants in 2002, has shown a lasting impact of the programme on individuals in three key areas: (Martin, 2003).

- **Understanding the 'big picture' or context of leadership:** Participants described the relevance of the learning they achieved in terms of it helping them to more fully understand and become involved in strategy and change management. This had greatly increased their confidence to practice as leaders, and to contribute to leadership agendas in their organisations.

  > "You lift your nose away from the grindstone! It is so easy to get drawn into fire-fighting and crises and the everyday demands and just never think beyond that. This was a chance to think about a different horizon."

- **Improving personal effectiveness:** Participants reported changing their behaviour to become more skilled in leadership, especially with respect to their ability to develop follower-ship and to build teams and alliances.

- **Networking and support:** Learning in a multi-agency and multi-professional environment greatly enriched the development programme, challenged thinking and narrow mind-sets and brought benefits through variety and new contacts.

> "The key was that this was multi-disciplinary – whether you are in service x or service y, PCT or mental health or acute, the problems are the same and they cross boundaries. This was about recognising that if we can understand each other then we can work together – sorting out care pathways, sorting out best value. Now we can share a language to talk to each other in."

The most significant impacts of the programmes in organisation development terms have been:

- **Changes in leadership behaviour** – 360° feedback has been highly significant in developing transformational leadership behaviours. Participants report using styles which enable greater empowerment of teams and service delivery staff through better delegation, more listening and idea-generation, and through encouraging more questioning and critical thinking about systems. 360° feedback gives a specific and evidenced focus to personal development. The whole experience of the development programme creates a context for working on this feedback which has both energised and supported participants to develop their own style and thinking. The experience was frequently described by participants as a much-valued investment in themselves.

    > "360° was awful, and excellent!"

    > "It forced me to look very closely at myself. If you've been around for a while you get to know the techniques and you can do it all without engaging the full set of emotions, but this pulled me up short, and it lead to a really fundamental change in my view of myself and my practice, all my interactions with the people I manage."

- **Networks:** The leadership development programme has created better links across organisational boundaries, a wider understanding of the realities and agendas of other service areas and an associated richer appreciation of others' issues. Participants described are using these networks to gather information and intelligence, and also to position themselves to contribute their leadership ideas and skills in new domains beyond traditional discipline or agency boundaries. Leaders emerged from the programme with a greater sense of issues across the delivery environment, mirrored in the make-up of their course group, and a shared language and approach to leadership.

- **Change management:** This is a key skill to which participants had radically altered their approach, making use of more empowering styles with their teams. They emphasised the importance of the skills of listening, building confidence and motivating others. Participants had been involved in service management changes, developing new service specifications and contributing to work groups, as well as implementing and working in new organisation structures. Their greater skill and confidence in handling change was a significant finding, as evidenced by leadership resources being successfully deployed on complex organisation agendas.

- **Thinking and leadership awareness:** Participants saw leadership as a set of skills which give permission to think, challenge, and make things happen. As well as creating their own identity as leaders, participants described a commitment to organisation development and to investment in the future development of individuals to deal with change and partnership.

  > "It was never spelled out how we should change – but it would have been deleterious had it been. There was an almost offhand feel about it – no exam, no dissertation, no pay rise, no fines. The whole attitude was 'you make of it what you will'. And I got the materials and the theory, the contacts, the chance to reflect, and you realise it really is up to you what you do with it."

Learning about the development of leaders in health and social care

1. **The multi-disciplinary and multi-agency ethos** that permeated the philosophy and practice of the programme created a learning environment which was both challenging and open, and, as it mirrored the delivery environment in which participants work, meant that realities across the spectrum of service domains were understood and actioned. It also significantly supported networking and created linkages which served leaders well in their work in change and partnership.

2. **360° feedback** was a vital stimulus to reflective practice, and challenged participants with the views of their immediate workplace

colleagues; 360° feedback is an acknowledged way of developing transformational behaviours, and a well-validated model which supports participants in making focused and evidenced developmental changes.

3. **A high-quality, flexible programme design** was needed, rather than either a pre-set or piecemeal approach. The Northumberland programme has received crucial support from a network of highly-experienced practitioners and excellent communicators to run interactive and diagnostic sessions which stimulate thinking and learning.

4. Consistency of developmental support and follow-through of learning was achieved through **skilled facilitation**. A team of facilitators worked with participants on the programme supporting Action Learning, and working closely with individuals to support them in their analysis of issues and in achieving development goals.

5. **Top management support** was needed to align the leadership development effort strategically with organisation transformation, visioning and re-structuring. Leadership development was a way of making an often-neglected link to the individuals who will make change happen and who need to exert leadership both through their own behaviour and through their confidence to act effectively across the most complex of service delivery environments. Chief Executives' support and sponsorship of the Northumberland programme was crucial in enabling such a significant investment in people as leaders in order to action their strategic vision of partnership for the benefit of the population they serve.

Conclusion

Leading a vision for change in Northumberland has been achieved through the dedication, commitment and inspiration of leaders from all the partner organisations. Developing and unlocking the creativity, talents and confidence of leaders through the leadership development programmes has been key to success. A leadership community and leadership learning network of over 200 leaders from all organisations continues and sustains the capacity and continuous self –directed development of leadership.

"Leadership Development has been an integral component of the organisational change programme in our health economy. Good leadership skills have never been more in demand in the NHS. Changes to all our working lives mean we need to motivate our teams to innovate and embrace new opportunities and become responsive to new agendas. This sort of change is not always comfortable and it needs skilful leaders to carry it forward. This is why we launched the Leadership Development Programme. It has enabled people to broaden their focus and to feel part of something that is organisation wide and even health economy wide.

In terms of building networks and making connections it has been invaluable. It helped us to build partnerships with other organisations. It helped us to wake up to the way the NHS and public service is generally changing, and how the organisation looks within that. It has facilitated significant change in service planning and delivery.

It has given people an array of different experiences in leadership and skills. Importantly it has challenged them. The programme unlocks ability, increases energy and confidence. Parochialism has reduced, job scope and ideas have increased, and peoples' ability to work on their own problems and issues is much improved. The 360° feedback was an excellent component that provided certainty in personal development.

The design allowed the provision of overall investment in people, in both time and space to learn and reflect. This eclectic learning was then followed by targeting specific needs helping individuals and teams develop. I have personally endorsed this programme and I am convinced that this investment in our people is the way forward to meet the demands of a very new kind of working world in healthcare."

Chief Executive's endorsement,
Northumberland health and social care organisations

"Without leadership systems fall apart – there is no decision making, no follow through. People just get stuck in doing the same thing day after day – and they will work hard and struggle with problems, but it makes no difference. If you have leadership, you make sure there are skills throughout the team to make change, you have freedom and time out to stop and think, to question, and the vision to do things differently."

References

Alimo-Metcalfe, B. & Alban-Metcalfe, J. (2003) "Stamp Of Greatness", *Health Service Journal* (26 June), pp 28–32.

Alimo Metcalfe, B. (2002) "Heaven can wait", *Health Service Journal* (12 October).

Alimo-Metcalfe, B. (1998) "The use of 360 degree feedback for developing leadership", *International Journal of Selection and Assessment*, Vol. 7, No. 1.

Antoniano, D. (1996) "Designing an effective 360 degree appraisal feedback process", *Organisational Dynamics* (Autumn), pp 24–38.

Cowie, W. (2003) *Leadership Development: Tees and North East Yorkshire NHS Trust.*

Foreman, A. (2002) *Leadership, Culture Change and Change Management,* Northumbria Healthcare NHS Trust.

Jarrold, K (1998) "A view from here: servants and leaders" in *Proceedings of the Fourth York Health Symposium,* Centre for Leadership Development, University of York.

Kolb, D. (1984) *Experiential Learning: Experience as the Source of Learning and Development,* New Jersey, Prentice-Hall.

Martin, S. (2003) *Evaluation of Leading a Vision for Change Development Programme.*

MRG (2000) *Leadership Effectiveness Analysis: Measures of Reliability and Validity,* Management Research Group, Munich.

Plsek, P. (2003) *Framework for the Leading Modernisation Programme.*

Stahr, H., Bulman, B. & Stead, M. (2000) *The Excellence Model in the Health Sector: Sharing Good Practice,* Chichester, Kingsham Press.

CHAPTER SIXTEEN

Leadership development within an acute NHS Trust

Jan Freer

> This chapter focuses on leadership development within an Acute NHS Trust. Leadership development is conceived of as a major component within a broader and more comprehensive organisation development strategy. In particular, the chapter focuses on the use of the LEO (Leading an Empowered Organisation) programme; associated supporting activity and on the application of Action Learning within the Trust.

Background

Calderdale and Huddersfield NHS Trust is an acute hospital Trust comprising two hospital buildings, one located in Halifax and the other in Huddersfield, about five miles apart. The Trust serves a population of about 500,000, covering two local authorities and has an income of just over £200 million with some 5,300 staff.

The Trust has experienced significant change in the two years to 2003 with the two former hospitals merging in April, 2001; only to lose their community and mental health services in April, 2002 to the three local Primary Care Trusts and the South West Yorkshire Mental Health Trust. Additionally, Calderdale also faced the challenge of merging three old hospitals onto one newly-built, privately-financed site, which became operational in June, 2001.

The original hospitals were fiercely owned by the people of the two towns and there was a history of rivalry and distrust between them. However, before 1997 and the arrival in Huddersfield of a new Chief Executive, the organisations had a similar culture and approach; both were fairly self-satisfied and parochial, paternalistic and proud of the services provided to their communities.

From a policy perspective, together with the new Chief Executive in Huddersfield, arrived a raft of Government reforms, demanding modernisation, standardisation, performance monitoring and transparent accountability. The introduction of the new standard frameworks for care – the National Service Frameworks (NSFs), along with the duty of quality of care enshrined in the new Clinical Governance arrangements, and the European Working Time Directive limiting junior doctors' hours, all meant that service collaboration, leading to Trust merger was inevitable. It was, however, not without some resistance that the two hospitals finally merged, led by the Huddersfield Chief Executive, supported by a mixed team of Calderdale and Huddersfield Executive Directors. Firstly, then, Huddersfield (as it changed in response to its new leader) and then Calderdale and Huddersfield emerged and evolved from two very different basic constituents.

Leadership development

The literature on leadership development is vast. What becomes clear in examining it, however, is that there is no real agreement on what makes a good leader; whether the qualities and attributes (whatever they are) are innate or can be learned; and if they can be learned, what the "magic formula" for that process might be. Faced with such a wealth of complexity and opinion and recognising that leadership development would need to be the rock upon which overall development of the organisation would have to be based, it was decided to keep the approach as simple as possible. There did, however, need to be an organisational approach. Within any organisation (and an NHS Trust is no exception) there are legions of people who are doing, or have done, further study, both for clinical and managerial purposes. Whatever the qualification, the course invariably involves a leadership module, in which all the different theories and approaches can be discussed and dissected. The result of this is an organisation full of "experts" on leadership, which is a heart-sinking situation for those unlucky enough to be tasked with the role of introducing leadership development activities! Discussing leadership is very similar to discussing Information Technology – everyone has a PC/laptop/personal organiser; can use different software packages and the Internet, and has spent many a happy hour in "PC World" – so they feel able to put the organisation's IT department right on any IT-related issues.

So, just as leadership is part of the core curriculum of innumerable courses, it crops up in many of the Trust's in-house training and development activities. It was felt that a common language and approach, shared across the Trust, would be a good building-block. The sort of organisation we had designed was devolved and clinically-led. That meant we were looking for leadership behaviours and attributes at *all* levels of the Trust. A key driver was to bridge the chasm between doctors and managers, doctors and nurses, allied health professionals (AHPs) and nurses, AHPs and managers, etc. The Trust chose to use a three-day programme known as "Leading an Empowered Organisation" (LEO), as the foundation for its leadership development approach. The reasons for this were varied. Firstly, the principles espoused by the programme were those that we were looking for our staff to embrace. They can be summarised as:

- Taking personal responsibility for one's actions
- Building and maintaining relationships with others
- Solving problems with a "can-do" approach, rather than problem-processing
- Encouraging risk taking to create new solutions and using failure as an opportunity for learning, not as an opportunity to punish
- Openly and assertively communicating and being clear about stating what needs to happen to be successful.

These principles are underpinned by a series of activities in the programme that allow participants to understand the material and to practice new skills and behaviours. The theoretical model used is Hersey and Blanchard's Situational Leadership (2000). This identifies both leadership *and* follower ship and recognises that depending upon the situation, leaders are also followers. This is a very powerful message for doctors and for others who achieve leadership roles by excelling as clinicians (or other functional specialists). Medical staff have to make decisions on the clinical management of patients, and even in fairly junior positions have to portray confidence and certainty to patients and to other staff to demonstrate their authority. In Hersey and Blanchard's model they are therefore in quadrant 4 as experts (see Figure 16.1).

However, when faced with new tasks, such as Clinical Directorship or Ward Management, clinicians become novices. Once such senior people

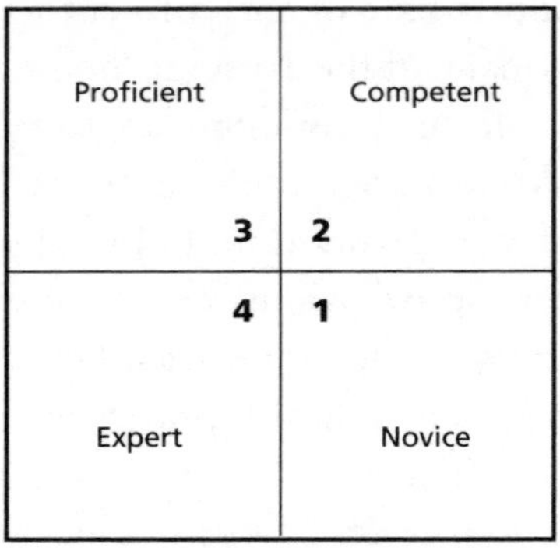

Proficient	Competent
3	**2**
4	**1**
Expert	Novice

Figure 16.1: Hersey & Blanchard's model of situational leadership

are given permission "not to know everything", and when it is recognised that, when discussing leader-follower roles, we are not necessarily talking about a hierarchical relationship, then they are much more open to personal development and supported learning.

A second key premise in the Hersey and Blanchard model is a related one – the role of leaders is to develop followers, and as a follower (depending upon where you are on the development path) you will need different styles from your leader. These styles are simply classified as Task Behaviour and Relationship Behaviour.

- *Task Behaviour* is defined as the extent to which the leader engages in spelling out the duties and responsibilities of an individual or group. When someone is new in post or new in the organisation, in order to succeed they need a high degree of direction.

- *Relationship Behaviour* is defined as the extent to which the leader engages in two-way or multi-way communication. This engagement includes listening, facilitating and supportive behaviours. When the stage of leadership growth in Figure 1 is combined with the style of leadership needed at each stage, this provides a useful model for all staff with leadership responsibilities, both to assess their own position and to ask for the right support to help them grow – and to assess their

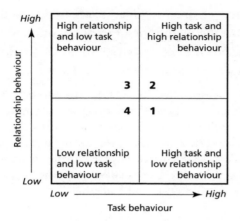

Figure 16.2: Leadership styles (Hersey & Blanchard)

follower's position and provide them individually with the right amount of direction and support. This is shown in Figure 16.2.

Finally, the content of the programme around the competencies of leaders is very relevant. LEO bases leadership competencies on Dorothy Del Bueno's model (1980). This identifies three domains in which all employees need to be skilful; the *technical* aspects of the job; those associated with *critical thinking*, and those associated with *interpersonal skills*. This model is shown in Figure 16.3.

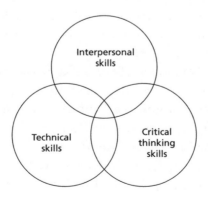

Figure 16.3: Del Bueno's leadership competencies

The importance of interpersonal relationships and behaviours is stressed, rather than the acquisition of technical or critical thinking skills. This is also reflected in Goleman's (1996) work on the importance of Emotional Intelligence in leaders where he states that:

> "I have found, however, that the most effective leaders are alike in one crucial way: they all have a high degree of what has come to be known as emotional intelligence. It's not that IQ and technical skills are irrelevant, they do matter, but mainly as "threshold capabilities"; that is, they are the entry level requirements for executive positions. But my research, along with other recent studies, clearly shows that emotional intelligence is the sine qua non of leadership".

Emotionally intelligent leaders are therefore the sort that we are looking to develop for the organisation.

Apart from organisational "fit", the Trust also chose LEO because it can be delivered under organisational licensing arrangements by the Trust's own staff via a "Train-the-Trainer" arrangement. This has two advantages. Firstly, it provides a cost-effective and sustainable solution to enable large numbers of staff to have the same experience; and secondly, using our own staff to facilitate the LEO programmes provides them with a development opportunity and fits our goal of combining the "day job" and development activity. Delivery of the programme by "real" managers and clinicians, rather than trainers, also gives the programme credibility, and the leadership examples they bring provide powerful learning tools.

LEO was first introduced into the Huddersfield Trust, endorsed by the Management Board in May, 2000. Initially, a general manager and the Head of OD became trainers, but over the 2001–2003 period the Trust has trained twelve facilitators (although some have left) and over five hundred staff have been "LEO-ed". A progress report, taken to the Trust Executive Board in November, 2002, reaffirmed organisational commitment. The approach has been recognised by all the Trust's external assessments and was commended by the Improving Working Lives (IWL) and Commission for Health Improvement (CHI) reports.

There is, however, a degree of ambivalence about this achievement. This is partly because the Trust Chief Executive has never really "signed-up" to the LEO programme. While there is no problem with the principles or content of the programme, there is antagonism to the concept of what is seen as a "sheep-dip" approach to leadership development. LEO has also been branded as a "nursing" programme, probably not helped by the NHS Leadership Centre commissioning 32,000 places for F & G grade nurses nationally, and, more recently, for 7,000 Allied Health Professionals and Health Care Scientists. These factors have been fairly significant obstacles to the introduction of LEO in the Trust, which have been addressed by working it through without drawing undue attention to it at Director level. While recognising the dangers of leadership fads and initiatives, for the moment LEO is seen as a useful arm of the Trust's leadership approach and helps to foster common messages and a corporate approach which is in line with our organisational culture, to a critical number of staff. Nonetheless, the Trust is prepared to "let go" of LEO when it has outlived its usefulness!

Supporting leadership development activities

Whilst LEO has been used as the "foundation programme", many other activities within the Trust also contribute to leadership development. Underpinning the Trust's approach are two major themes. The first is building internal capacity and capability for organisational development and the second is, wherever possible, to work with a recognised academic partner to provide weight and credibility.

A key academic partner is the Centre for the Development of Healthcare Policy and Practice (CDHPP) at the University of Leeds. Their approach is one of "Training-the-Trainers" and building-up the capacity and skills in the organisations with which they work to deliver their products in-house using the local leadership development community. This approach fits well with our philosophy and, as well as the LEO programme, the Trust partners with them to provide the following:

- *Leadership Effectiveness Analysis*™ *(LEA)* – A 360° diagnostic and development tool.
- *Flexible Thinking* – A programme that presents and promotes practical lateral-thinking and creativity skills such as "Mind Mapping", "Six Thinking Hats", etc.
- *Entrepreneurship* – A programme that develops individuals' negotiating and communication skills, giving them confidence to promote their skills and services.

- *Practice Development Units* – A framework for improving multi-disciplinary team-based services in clinical areas considering standard-setting, patient involvement, benchmarking, assessment and development.

These programmes have common elements and themes. The Trust has a number of accredited trainers and presenters within the organisation from both clinical and managerial backgrounds, who are supported and quality-assured by Leeds University.

Action Learning

In earlier work in the pre-merger, Huddersfield Trust OD Strategy a primary responsibility was to introduce Action Learning in association with the Revans Institute for Action Learning and Research at the University of Salford. The driver for this was the then recently-appointed Chief Executive whose personal history with the Revans Institute provided a company of friends and colleagues for ongoing support for people like herself at senior levels in healthcare organisations. The Chief Executive wanted to bring those benefits into the Trust and to encourage that sense of learning and fellowship that she found so valuable. This was a challenge, given the prevailing culture in the Trust. There was little or no understanding of organisational development; the organisation in general was task-focused, fairly complacent and non-reflective. It was also narrowly-focused in professional and developmental "silos". People worked in their functional areas, taking little personal responsibility for how changes in their area might impact on the organisation as a whole.

Supporting the development of the new approach was the Trust's external OD adviser who introduced the importance of working "outside the box" and making corporate as well as functional contributions. "Project-Based Working" became one of the labels for changing practice, and because projects are task-based and with measurable outcomes, this was something the Trust could endorse. There was concern that Action Learning would not be met with the same level of enthusiasm, and yet, unlike Project-Based Working, there was a strong belief that building Action Learning into the fabric of organisational life could make a tangible difference to us. The approach adopted was intuitive and empirical.

Seven projects were initiated, all endorsed as critical to the success of the organisation and sponsored by members of the Executive Board, with the project leads forming an Action Learning set supported by the Revans Institute. The "tone" adopted at this stage was businesslike and formal with a greater emphasis on education and progress, rather than on learning and development.

That first Action Learning set in Huddersfield, with its seven project leaders, built a firm foundation for its continuation into Calderdale and Huddersfield Trust. In December, 2001 a proposal to continue and to extend the programme was agreed at the Trust Management Board. This included two additional features. Firstly, the ability of set members to register with the Revans Institute for a higher qualification, and secondly, the use of the original set members as set advisers to new sets, whilst at the same time maintaining their original set membership to help guide and quality assure their progress and development as set advisers. This model (reproduced below in Figure 16.4) fulfils the two key criteria of building the Trust's internal capacity and creating academic links.

A number of sets were developed in line with this model and a progress report was presented to the Trust Executive Board eight months later describing six Action Learning sets with thirty eight participants. This strand of activity has been both pleasing and disappointing. The pleasure is associated with the thirty-eight participants, and the level of interest and engagement that Action Learning has engendered in the Trust. There are however, two particular disappointments. Firstly, having set the standard of set adviser as someone who has been involved with the Revans Institute approach to Action Learning, we have been unable to meet the demand for Action Learning sets from this resource. Secondly, pivotal to the strategy was a set comprising the senior medical personnel in the Trust – the three Medical directors and the four Divisional Directors. Because there was pressure to introduce this, there was an equal and opposite reaction, and the set failed to develop. This example from the top was important both because the would-be set members were clinicians (and doctors engaging in Action Learning is a powerful tool for change) and also because as senior members of the Trust Executive, their participation gives a strong message about the importance of learning and meeting together on a regular basis to everyone else in the organisation. The Chief Executive's approach was, however, philosophical – Action Learning

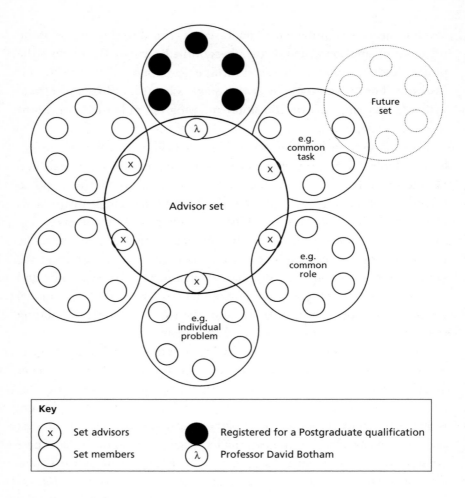

Figure 16.4: Action Learning in the Trust

doesn't suit everyone, nor was it ever meant to be a compulsory corporate tool for development.

Reviewing the progress of Action Learning, it is fair to say that, over time, the emphasis has gradually changed as the organisation has become more accustomed to looking at itself more critically and has developed a greater level of self-awareness. The task and the development focus are now both equally acceptable. Mentioning learning no longer creates raised eyebrows and an embarrassed cough. This kind of change happens imperceptibly and is difficult or even impossible to prove or to measure.

Conclusion

In summary, the Trust's leadership development stream of activity aims to create emotionally intelligent leaders who promote and exemplify the learning organisation (Pedler *et al.*, 1991). Different threads are contained in the Trust's structure, its culture and in leadership development, and there is some evidence that they are beginning to weave together and to produce an encouraging picture. The recent Commission for Health Improvement Report included the following statement:

> "The Trust has an inclusive, strong and devolved leadership. There is an open learning culture where mistakes and issues of poor performance are handled in a responsible way and staff are encouraged to develop their skills. Although the clinical management arrangements are still new, the Trust is a well managed organisation and clinicians and managers are working well together."

CHI, 2002

References

CHI (2002) *Clinical Governance Review: Calderdale and Huddersfield NHS Trust,* London, Commission for Health Improvement.

Del Bueno, D., Barker, J. & Christmyer, L. (1980) "Implementing a competency-based orientation program", *Nurse Educator*, May/June, pp. 16–20.

Goleman, D. (1988) "What makes a leader?", *Harvard Business Review*, November–December.

Hersey, P., Blanchard, K. & Johnson, D.(2000) *Management of Organisational Behaviour: Leading Human Resources*, 8th ed., NJ, Prentice Hall.

CHAPTER SEVENTEEN

From small acorns large oak trees grow: a story of whole systems leadership

Denise Houghton

"This story is recommended to the reader as one of demonstrating real strength, great vision and organisational teamwork on a grand scale. Not one person's leadership achievement, but that of the collective many, that made up the Rochdale Healthcare NHS Trust."

Introduction

The beginning of this journey started out as a relatively simple idea, that being to identify a whole systems accreditation system and to navigate an average-sized NHS Trust in England through the process.

Following an extensive global search the Magnet framework was identified as being the most suitable (and yet most challenging) framework available. It was here that the Magnet journey started, building on a very successful model of leadership that was already demonstrating positive change in terms of both the service and clinical practice, through a devolved system of decision-making and staff empowerment.

This chapter presents to the reader a very practical example of how leadership, learning and education can turn an organisation into a world-class leader, from a position of being an average organisation in the NHS – to become one of a prestigious few who had achieved recognition for excellence across a whole system of service provision. And more importantly, in this context, empowering clinicians to take charge of their own agenda though a process of engagement and feedback presented to service leaders, practitioners and the whole organisation.

This chapter offers the story of this accreditation – the stages of evolution the organisation went through to achieve its application; the changes faced along the way and the challenges that those have presented to the organisation. The evidence identifies the organisation's real strengths, while at the same time as articulating real weaknesses. However, accreditation in this context is viewed as a destination not to be achieved at the first cross roads, but to be embraced as part of a continuous journey of quality improvement.

In becoming leaders of change and exploring new horizons the journey of quality improvement took this particular organisation to the point of the end of the last century. As well as being a real privilege, it also presented considerable challenges. Not only was the concept of whole systems accreditation new, and indeed unknown, territory in the NHS in England, but the Trust had made a decision to experiment with a model which was at the time part of (and had been created for) a very different healthcare system.

In taking the lead with such an initiative, Rochdale saw itself leading a national project in the global field. With that in mind, one of the additional challenges has been to share findings on a very regular basis both in the formal sense (through conferences and major seminars) but also through developing international networks and receiving visitors who wished to examine and question that progress along the way. At the beginning of this journey Magnet was a United States phenomenon, whereas it is now a professional validation tool of international comparisons.

The context

Rochdale .is an old Lancashire mill town, sitting at the bottom of the Northern Pennines on the border of Lancashire and Yorkshire. The population is around 220,000, with a 20% ethnic minority population mainly originating from the Indian sub-continent. This is not a wealthy locale. The economy had suffered from the economic changes of the twentieth century and still bears the scars of the cotton industry's demise. However, investment – through the area being identified as a regeneration area (Single Regeneration Budget or SRB) and Health Action Zone (HAZ), has brought a degree of movement and growth into the area.

A consequence of this poor economic environment is a negative profile of health, when set against a comparative national profile. The area has the highest national Standard Mortality Rates (SMRs) for coronary heart disease, diabetes and respiratory illness. Whilst the neonatal mortality rate is good compared to the national profile, Rochdale babies are born meeting the definition of low birth weight. Such a health profile presents considerable challenges to the local health economy.

Rochdale Healthcare NHS Trust, prior to its merger into the Pennine Acute Hospitals NHS Trust, was an integrated healthcare organisation offering a full portfolio of services to the local population. Embraced within its business portfolio were the directorates of medicine, surgery, maternal and child health, community and learning disabilities and mental health. For the purposes of the Magnet application it is important to point out that the success of this application meant that it was the first time that such clinical services of midwifery, learning disability and community nursing had been reviewed through the Magnet process. This was further evidence that the Magnet framework could be applied in any healthcare context.

The nursing contribution

The strategic direction for nursing in Rochdale was based on a foundation of leadership and empowerment, this being realised through the development of a leadership culture based on a model of Shared Governance (Williamson & Petts, 2000; Edmonstone, 2003) and devolved decision-making. Nursing was not seen to be functioning separately but was being enabled to make a corporate contribution. Nurses and nursing shared the corporate agenda.

Through the Shared Governance council structure nurses and therapists were responsible for leading, developing and changing practice. It was through this very important vehicle that the journey towards accreditation was achieved. Recognition along the way in this journey came through the mental health directorate achieving Practice Development Unit (PDU) status through an accreditation process for PDUs run by the Centre for the Development of Healthcare Policy & Practice at Leeds University, and the Diabetic centre achieving the Government's Charter

Mark – a national award based on patient recommendation and external validation.

Through encouraging, nurses and therapists to innovate and lead the organisation could demonstrate real evidence in changing roles and responsibilities for various practitioners within care teams. The appointment of nurse consultants and other key nursing roles, some of them working within a career ladder framework, enabled practice capability to continue to move forward. The experience of Rochdale in developing this area also informed the work by the Department of Health's Human Resources Directorate on the notion of the "skills escalator". Such workforce redesign initiatives were also very much supported by the Greater Manchester Workforce Development Confederation – such was the scale of innovation and change back in the late nineties. One visitor to Rochdale observed that the Trust "Had more pilots than Gatwick Airport!" This illustrates the point that empowering individuals with sufficient authority automatically drives the organisation in a direction that pursues excellence. It is not an objective that has to be forced.

Clearly, in order to achieve increased capability sound educational systems need to be in place. Practice educator posts were introduced into the clinical areas to work with and alongside nurses in practice. The objective was to develop skills and to improve standards of care.

Practitioners were encouraged to underpin their practice with the appropriate evidence. All clinicians should have at their disposal appropriate access to the relevant clinical evidence bases to guide and inform their clinical work. The basic tools of clinical practice were thus made available to them. This added to the empowerment process and generated a culture of staff feeling valued for the contribution they had to make.

The Magnet philosophy works on the basis that if the organisation looks after its clinical staff, the staff in turn care more effectively for patients and patient outcomes are seen to improve. This has been demonstrated time and time again though the Rochdale experience.

Why pursue accreditation?

The strategic context surrounding healthcare systems in the NHS in England in the late 1990s and the early years of the 21st century had changed to such an extent that *not* to begin to consider accreditation would have been short-sighted. The developing and presenting policy framework in support of modernising the NHS was a significant driver in moving the debate forward. The emerging clinical quality agenda was set to facilitate an overall improvement in clinical performance – indeed, in how clinicians behaved.

The National Institute for Clinical Excellence (NICE) was looking at developing the evidence base of clinical practice and facilitating the development of national guidance on key healthcare practices and the whole system was being monitored by the then Commission for Health Improvement (CHI), now known as the Commission for Health Improvement, Audit and Inspection (CHAI). The national Human Resource strategy was beginning to emerge on the agenda as a framework supporting significant change and the national Strategy for Nursing "Making a Difference" (DoH, 1999) were all set to drive the agenda forward, in terms of defining what was meant by good and excellent practice and the environment in which care was delivered.

Whilst the Rochdale Healthcare NHS Trust had an obligation (and indeed a commitment) to deliver on the national policy agenda, there were also several local drivers that highlighted the need for practice systems to be recognised through a formal framework.

Firstly, the organisation was committed to improving professional practice through its commitment to ongoing professional education. Secondly, the organisation was committed to being a good employer of professional staff. Thirdly, there was a demonstrated desire to develop a culture based on shared leadership principles and a devolved model of decision-making. Fourthly (and perhaps the most pressing issue), was the need for the whole organisation to become involved in the re-configuration process going on in the local health economy. The final key point was that to survive in a future healthcare system the Trust had to recruit the best staff available. To do so meant that Rochdale had to attract a workforce which was committed to delivering the organisational mission in a whole new environment – a workforce which desired quality in the care delivered and which was educated to delivering care in that way.

Delivering the organisation to the point of accreditation

The challenge of leading an "average" healthcare organisation to the point of achieving whole systems accreditation should not be underestimated. It was very much part of an overall five-year strategy which was based primarily on leadership development, thus enabling the organisation to take responsibility for the change agenda. Through being given the authority individuals were primed to deliver the overall challenge – and in this case rose to the challenge in hand.

The five-year plan was viewed very much as a journey of ongoing development. The point had long been recognised that once the stage of recognised quality improvement had been achieved, then a system of recognition and accreditation would be introduced.

The system chosen happened to be American for the reasons previously mentioned. As a consequence, it was felt by the leadership in Rochdale that the framework should be piloted. An agreement was reached with the American Nurses' Credentialing Centre (ANCC) to support a two-year pilot, which would explore the following hypothesis:

> "Is the Magnet framework transferable to the NHS and the European healthcare market?"

A management framework for the pilot followed the Projects In Controlled Environments (PRINCE) methodology. There are several points worth making with regard to the pilot which delivered significant learning through the experience gained.

Firstly, a manager was recruited to lead the initiative and the appointment was made from outside the organisation, as this was felt to be good practice. As it turned out, the leadership of such a challenging initiative was too complex for the individual concerned. Following his departure a very different approach was agreed. That was for a shared approach between the Director of Nursing, the Deputy Director of Nursing and the Senior Nurse (Practice Development).

The difficulties of making an external appointment to such an initiative reflect the importance of organisational intelligence. Appreciation of organisational networks and the local culture clearly enable project managers to 'hit the ground running'.

A second point related to having a real understanding of the Magnet framework and of the people who led its administration in the ANCC.

Although an internationally-based induction programme had been offered, this was not sufficient to adequately support the external appointee.

A third point was around the membership of the project board. As with all project boards the prime purpose was to provide strategic leadership and support to the initiative. The membership of the board reflected the fact that this was viewed as an international experiment. The project had the privilege of being supported by several great and significant names in international nurse leadership and policy and this meant that international promotion of the project was kept at a very high profile. Membership also reflected all the key organisational stakeholders – the ANCC, the Royal College of Nursing (RCN), the Department of Health (DoH), and the key academic centres with the designated academic leads present around the table.

Fourthly, was the recruitment and appointment of 70 Magnet champions who represented each clinical area across the Trust. Their prime purpose was to provide leadership to local teams and to be the main point of communication; but to also be given the authority to lead the necessary changes that were required to develop practice to the required standard. They were also the main point for the collection of evidence, which would ultimately be sent for validation by the ANCC Commission – the accrediting body of the Magnet Programme.

The fifth point well worth mentioning here is that throughout the whole process there was continuous review of the journey and celebration along the way. This contributed to the profile of the initiative within the organisation and maintained motivation and organisational interest at a very high level. Although it was exceptionally challenging and very hard work it was also seen to be great fun, good team building and, more importantly, became very much part of the organisational memory. This has been particularly important now that the organisation has merged, and has lost its original identity.

The application process

One of the key benefits of the Magnet application process is that learning and organisational growth continues. This is as a consequence of the great number of opportunities that individuals have to lead the many and varied activities that go to achieve the end result. It was interesting to observe that throughout the project the view was that it did not matter if accreditation was not achieved. What was important was the learning that was gained along the way. The organisation flourished, and the process influenced all personnel, from clinical staff through to domestic and catering staff.

The collection of evidence was coordinated through the Magnet champions. There were many and interesting approaches adopted. For example, to help ease the burden of their work the Learning Disabilities service negotiated a sponsorship by a soft drinks company who produce the drink "Iron Brew". This was chosen to illustrate a connection with Magnet, and metal. The company provided refreshments for the groups during their deliberations and evidence-collecting sessions.

This same group also chose to produce a video, which was designed to tell the Magnet story to learning disabled clients. It was appropriately called "Alice in Magnet Land", and was produced in conjunction with the local sixth form college.

The Magnet accreditation process works along a conceptual process of what would be called in the UK "triangulation", but which American colleagues refer to as *Clarification*, *Amplification* and *Verification*. The submission of evidence supports this process through submission of the evidence and assessment at two levels – firstly, at the standard of the American Nurses Association, and secondly, against the Magnet standards of excellence. The stages of amplification and verification are met through site visits by the accreditation teams, followed by submission of the accreditation team's report to the Commission, supported by a peer review system of votes based upon an overall assessment of the evidence against standards.

Lessons learnt from the pilot

The pilot was to have lasted two years. However, after eighteen months it was felt by the project board that there was sufficient evidence to continue as an applicant site. Whilst the project board recommended this it was the organisation which made the decision to become a formal applicant. The decision was also influenced by the fact that the merger was felt to be less than twelve months away and the opportunity would then be lost.

The most challenging part of the whole process was the interpretation of the American language and clinical terms. The Magnet framework is transferable internationally. However, the difference in language between the health systems in question poses a long-term challenge for the ANCC if this is to be seen as a global phenomenon. This language debate continues almost two years after Rochdale's achievement was recognised.

The cost of application is expensive and could be seen as prohibitive to publicly-funded organisations like the NHS. The cost-benefits of Magnet accreditation are currently being evaluated by Professor James Buchan of Queen Margaret University College on behalf of the Department of Health.

It was important that there was also some ongoing evaluation of the project and tracking of the impact on the organisation. The evaluation was undertaken, by a team from St Martins College, Lancaster University, (Cook and Bologue, 2003).

Life after accreditation

Throughout the life of the project and subsequent application process there was a commitment by the project team to share learning both through encouraging site visits (which added to the empowerment of both patients and staff) and also through involving the media and presenting at conferences.

The visits became so popular that the site now hosts a series of open days, which involve staff taking centre-stage, continuing to build their confidence and profile.

The most significant thing to have subsequently happened to Rochdale was an acute services merger with three other similar-sized organisations to create the largest acute healthcare provider in the country. Whilst this has been very threatening and challenging for many it has also been interesting to observe the staff in Rochdale. The nursing staff, as a consequence of their level of earned autonomy, have coped well with the change in organisational leadership, taking on the mantle of site leadership. This has been observed and commented on many times over by new people coming into the new Trust. In particular, the new chief executive viewed the nurses in Rochdale as different. They are, of course, Magnet nurses!

As with any organisational accreditation process there is continuous monitoring. This is through an annual reporting and monitoring system administered by the ANCC Commission.

Without doubt the achievement of Magnet accreditation has improved the sites' recruitment and retention capability. Other notable workforce achievements are in relation to staff sickness and absence and staff opinion and morale.

Clinical outcomes have continued to improve, with a demonstrated improvement in complaints, with both in a reduction of numbers and in complexity.

In the summer following Magnet accreditation the previous Rochdale NHS Trust achieved a 3-star rating in the NHS performance league tables – clearly an achievement influenced by the Magnet journey.

The previously-mentioned Trust merger in bringing with it massive organisational change and has influenced the future positioning of the Rochdale site, both in terms of the current position and of the re-accreditation process.

So, where to next? Clearly, there is a commitment from the staff in Rochdale and the new Trust to maintaining Magnet recognition. There is equally, a vision which would see the whole of the Pennine Acute Hospitals NHS Trust experience the Magnet journey and ultimately accreditation. At this point the journey is just beginning, and the future looks awesome!

In concluding this chapter, I would reflect that such a journey cannot be achieved by one individual. Transformational leadership in this context is the story of many individuals coming together to share the same goals and ultimate vision. From the size of an acorn to that of an old oak tree!

Acknowledgements

These are due to Nicola Nicholls and Steve Taylor and to the many colleagues that made such an awesome vision a reality. A special acknowledgement goes to Robert Clegg. Without his leadership and support, as the previous Chief Executive, none of this would have been possible.

References

Balogh, R., Cook, M. & Smith, H. (2003) *Attracting Evidence for Magnet Accreditation: the First Experience of Attempting and Gaining Magnet Accreditation Outside the USA at Rochdale Healthcare NHS Trust*, St Martin's College, University of Lancaster.

DoH (1999) *Making a Difference: Strengthening the Nursing, Midwifery and Health Visiting Contribution to Health and Healthcare*, London, Department of Health.

Edmonstone, J. (2003) *Shared Governance: Making it Happen*, Chichester, Kingsham Press.

Williamson, T. & Petts, S. (2000) *Shared Governance Survey Report: Evaluation of the Implementation of Shared Governance in an Integrated NHS Trust*, University of Salford/Rochdale Healthcare NHS Trust.

CHAPTER EIGHTEEN

Using Rich Pictures to promote team leadership

Christina Edwards

> "Adapt or perish, now as ever, is nature's inexorable imperative"
>
> H.G. Wells

Public services are complex organisations – especially the NHS, where different professions have different influence and power bases. In order to deliver services, managers and clinical staff often have to interact and liaise with many other organisations, both statutory and voluntary. The direction of travel and policy agenda is determined by Government, and the Service is not only constantly in the public eye, but is subject to scrutiny by the media and now through statute by local authorities.

The delivery of care by autonomous professionals who exercise their professional judgement was, historically, always the case. Increasingly with the development of clinical pathways, managed clinical networks, the National Service Frameworks and other evaluation approaches, including audit within clinical governance, the scene is changing even more quickly.

Most of the work of the NHS is delivered by teams, with very little of it delivered by individuals. Certainly an individual hospital consultant will see a patient (or a patient and his/her carer) but with him (and behind him) there is a comprehensive team of nurses, allied health professionals, caterers, receptionists and other members of the professional and support team. Much has been written about multi-disciplinary and multi-professional team development and about the importance of team working. Recently a research study by Aston Business School (West, 2002) demonstrated a clear link between effective team-working and lower patient mortality.

The challenge is getting teams to acknowledge the issues that are most pertinent, prioritising them and taking action in order to become a more competent team. This can improve the service and the management or the level of care given to patients. In my own experience, the more senior the team the more they may feel threatened by facing-up to individual problems and issues, personality clashes or frustrations that have an impact on them as an individual, but also on the team and its ability to work effectively. The work which the National Clinical Governance Team has been doing through the Clinical Governance Development Programme has shown clearly that encouraging team-working enhances governance, increases job satisfaction and improves service delivery.

Soft System Methodology (SSM), originally developed by Checkland (Checkland, 1981), and subsequently further elaborated (Checkland and Scholes, 1990), forms a seven-stage model comprising a complete set of actions which provide guidelines for systems improvement.

> "The methodology is a means of guiding the tackling of real world situations which are perceived as problematical for some of the time by at least one member of the situation"
>
> Davies and Leddington, 1991

An element of SSM is the use of "Rich Pictures". As Checkland & Scholes state – "A characteristic of fluent users of SSM is that they will be observed throughout the work drawing pictures and diagrams as well as taking notes and writing prose. The reason for this is that human affairs reveal a rich moving pageant of relationships, and pictures are a better means for recording relationships and connections than is linear prose."

When problems present themselves in a team situation, or where a new service or a change of service is planned, it is helpful to find a way to enable all the players to participate in both interpreting what the issues are, but also to find ways of working through the hurdles which block successful outcomes from taking place.

It has been suggested that "The methodology is concerned with getting from finding-out about a problem situation to taking action to improve it… You do this by building a cartoon-type representation of it which is called, in the jargon of the approach, a Rich Picture"(Naughton, 1984).

During the past few years I have been able to use this part of the SSM approach to enable both managerial and clinical teams to recognise the situation they find themselves in; to vision the future as it could be, and then to work through how they as a team can make improvements. It enables them to recognise unhelpful behaviours and the work which individuals and the team can do in order to improve. It is very important, when using this methodology, that the leader/manager/senior person in the team is happy, or at least prepared, to hear feedback on the issues that the team recognise need changing – which includes their leadership, but also how the team works together. It is important that wherever possible this person is part of the planning process and knows what may occur. Rich Pictures can identify problem situations in an often more helpful and less threatening way than a textual description. They can convey a more meaningful picture of the situation by explaining the system, behaviours and relationships contained within the problem, for example, ill-defined, fuzzy, value-laden, "wicked" political problems.

Rich Pictures uses symbolism to represent situations and much of what occurs in organisations is symbolic (Hirscheim and Newman, 1991). Happenings which others would see as unimportant, trivial or as organisational rituals can have a greater impact on people and teams working productively than their face value would suggest. We need ways to understand why these particular issues have a great symbolic significance to this particular organisation or part of it.

Rich Pictures are a type of metaphor. The Pictures simplify experiences, emotions and behaviours which are too complex and muddled to describe in language alone. So the Pictures need to describe the situation through demonstrating human activity and situations, and such things as power-play and political undertones. Checkland (1981) suggests the use of the Mnemonic CATWOE to define the production of the Pictures i.e. Customers, Actors, Transformation, Owners, Weltanscharung (Worldview) and Environment.

So, in a situation involving healthcare organisations or teams **CATWOE** could be demonstrated by:

- Patients/clients/carers as *Customers*
- Staff as *Actors*
- The need to improve team-working as *Transformation*

- The team needing to improve performance, quantity or quality of working in order to give better service or added value being a worthwhile thing to do as *Weltanschauung* (World-view).
- Those who can stop the system operating (the public or politicians for instance) – *Owners*
- The constraints, resources, silo working, difficult relationships, etc as *Environment*

With colleagues I have used the methodology on a number of occasions with different groups – an Executive Team of a large Community and Acute Trust; teams of senior nurses; and latterly with teams of hospital consultants. It is important that the work is followed through and that participants who have been able to describe not only the present situation but the future as they would like it to be, have support, guidance and development where necessary to work through the journey that together they need to take to meet their aspirations and goals. What could be a negative result of the work would be when the team sees the result of their work having no impact on the service. It would also be negative for the team to see no commitment or action to change the direction of travel or behaviour of the team and its leadership. It is extremely important to have some early "first wins" from the work so that the participants feel that notice is being taken of their suggestions and that there is support in order for them to deliver improvement.

In the first exercise with an Executive Team in a large Acute Trust and Community NHS, we divided the Executive Group, clinical directors and others into two groups who were then asked to draw the organisation as they thought it was presently "warts and all". They were encouraged to use similes for the drawings. One group used the fast food industry to represent the different organisations, with Ronald MacDonald as head of the organisation sitting on top of a castle shooting arrows at colleague organisations such as. GP fund-holders and Social Services. These stakeholder organisations were also represented by other fast food chains (see Figure 18.1).

I have found that the idea behind using Pictures (which represent people, organisations, and situations) helpful. There is safety in using humour but also imagination to explain the situation which the organisation and individuals find themselves in.

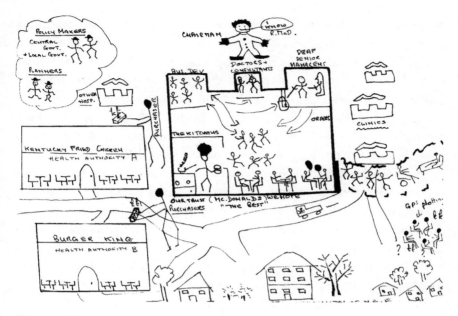

Figure 18.1

Another team drew a ship representing their own organisation, a sea in which there were many sharks and small boats and islands representing the different organisations that the Trust had to work with. A shark infested sea was how they viewed the surroundings of their own organisation.

The Chief Executive, who had been briefed and prepared, and was fully supportive and engaged in the exercise, was both surprised and provoked by the pictures the teams drew. He stated that he had no idea of the issues and concerns that underpinned the working relationships and concerns of his top team. It gave him a clearer idea of the work that the team, with himself at the helm, had to do to in order to ensure that people felt recognised and valued, and that better use was made of individual talents and experience to plan and develop services.

Some of the drawings can be humorous, but they can also be violent, uncomfortable, or sad. The feelings of the team and the agreement between them must be clearly set out in the sketch. It is then important to ask somebody to feedback on behalf of the group. That individual should be happy to illustrate the meanings as well as the obvious issues presented in the drawing. With good feedback the two or three teams can develop understanding and agreement about the key themes coming out of the drawings and which are the important issues that need to be dealt with. After feedback and discussion the group or groups can draw the future as they would like it to be. You can allow people to be as imaginative and as "off the wall" as they want to be, but to know when they need feedback on their hopes and vision for the future they should suggest a possible pathway to many of the objectives that they illustrate.

Again feedback is crucially important and the group needs to nominate its own volunteer to do this, but also to support them in doing this (sometimes challenging) task. This can be quite a lengthy process. For the drawing you need at least 45 minutes for the group to settle down together and feel brave and imaginative. The second drawing can be done in about 30 minutes but the important period is the feedback, both in the middle and then after the second drawing.

Some groups prefer to illustrate the problem by series of boxes, lines, triangles, creating a more theoretical model rather than drawing a picture. Each is totally acceptable and must be based on the group's own preferences (Figure 18.2). The final session is to draw together themes, acknowledging both the positives and the negatives and the hurdles and to construct the journey and the messages, which come out of the session, and which the group agrees can and should be taken forward in the future.

Recent sessions using Rich Pictures were with a hospital consultant specialist team who had been subject to an external review of the service. The Trust in which they worked was made up of two hospitals some miles apart and which had merged in recent years. As with many other mergers, the cultures of the two organisations were very different and concerns had been expressed regarding the split speciality and different working practices, workloads and commitment of the clinical staff. Morale was low and some members of the team felt extremely vulnerable. Asked to do some team development, my colleague and I pondered on the best and most constructive and least threatening way to help problems and challenges to emerge.

In the first instance I met with each individual consultant to allow them to express their views, but also to assure them that the session would

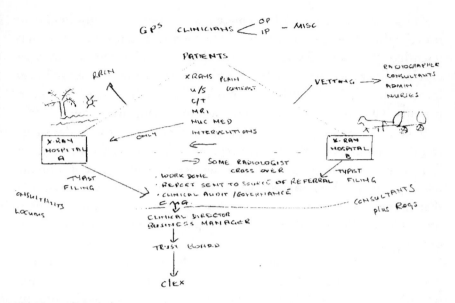

Figure 18.2

be enjoyable and non-threatening and that they would have the choice to participate as much or as little as they individually wished.

The result was a positive session, attended by all but one of the consultants, and the pictures drawn ranged from amusing and provocative, to serious and system-like. The feedback from each of the three groups on the present situation was open and honest, and demonstrated similar themes from each. The non-attendee was followed up with a letter and feedback about the outcome of the session.

The next drawings/illustrations of where they wanted to go and what their vision for the future shape, content and deliverables of the service they wished to provide was equally thoughtful and positive. Again the feedback and the list of agreement for actions by themselves and the team and requests to top management for support were agreed between them.

When we suggested several alternatives for the next session, which included meeting teams on the two separate sites, there was immediate disagreement with this plan. They stated "We wish to become a united team, working as one across both sites, so you must meet us together not separately."

The second session included representatives from the multidisciplinary team, and feedback to the Clinical Director and Executive Director representing the Chief Executive. They had identified further work to develop the service, but they felt that they were now acknowledged as an important, crucial speciality to modernise and improve services to patients. They also reported a willingness to develop and change.

It needs to be stressed that both the facilitator and the leader of the team(s) need to be confident and prepared to hear and deal with uncomfortable or difficult issues, both of a managerial nature, but also on any relationship or behavioural problems that are presented. It is also crucial that thought has been given about how support and guidance will be offered to individuals who may still feel side-lined or unhappy, at the end of this process.

The main objectives should be to make the process a positive and productive exercise and good preparation is the key. For instance, in a situation where members of the team may be damaged or vulnerable, jumping in to do a Rich Picture event can prove more harmful than helpful. In these cases meeting all the individual members of the team who will participate on a one-to-one basis before the event can be helpful to the facilitator and staff members. This will give an opportunity for individuals to express their concerns, worries or fears about opening-up difficult issues. They can be assured that the pictures are a way of conveying difficult messages in a light-hearted and corporate manner, rather than individuals being blamed. It also gives the facilitator the chance to put more anxious people in teams where they will be supported and helped to share issues.

Corporate (team or organisation) decline generally does not stem from a single factor; it results from an accumulation of decisions, actions, and commitments that became entangled in self-perpetuating workplace dynamics. Secrecy, blame, isolation, avoidance, lack of respect, and feelings of helplessness create a culture that makes an already bad situation worse. (Kanter, 2003).

The following are some helpful suggestions as to how a Rich Picture can be constructed:

1. Think of the elements of the situation you wish to illustrate in the picture and "draw" them using symbols, stick people or caricatures.

2. Put in structures such as buildings, equipment or symbols of these.
3. Demonstrate things that are changing or activities that take place.
4. Give impressions of interactions or organisational climate or culture.
5. Do not represent the situation as systems but use symbols.
6. Include hard factual data if you wish and soft subjective information too.
7. Demonstrate social roles which are meaningful to the team.
8. Annotate where helpful but keep brief.
9. Include all the players including yourself if appropriate.
10. Give a descriptive title to the picture.
11. The pictures are personal to the group; can be shared only if felt to be useful and agreement has been reached but messages and themes are currency to share with the wider team and other stakeholders for action to take place and be supported.

Using Rich Pictures can be a helpful and positive way of opening up difficult problem situations and help build team-working. They can assist in identifying work with both a developmental and managerial focus which can deliver a way to improve working systems in order to enhance services directly or indirectly for customers (our patients) and to enhance the working lives of our staff.

References

Checkland, P. (1981) *Systems Thinking, Systems Practice*, Chichester, Wiley.

Checkland, P. & Scholes, J. (1990) *Soft Systems Methodology in Action*, Chichester, Wiley.

Cullen, R., Nicholls, S. & Halligan, A. (2001) "Measurement to demonstrate success", *British Journal of Clinical Governance*, Vol. 6, No. 4, pp 273–278.

Cullen, R., Nicholls, S. & Halligan, A. (2000) "NHS support team: reviewing a service – discovering the unwritten roles", *British Journal of Clinical Governance*, Vol. 5, No. 4, pp 233–239.

Davies, L & Leddington, P. (1991) *Information in Action*, London, MacMillan Information Systems Series.

Hirschheim, R & Newman, M. (1991) "Symbolism and information system development: myth, metaphor and magic", *Information Systems Research*, Vol. 2, No. 1, pp 29–62.

Kanter, R (2003) "Leadership and the psychology of turnarounds", *Harvard Business Review* (June), pp 59–67.

Nicholls, S., Cullen, R. & Halligan, A. (2001) "Clinical governance …after the review – what next?: agreement and implementation", *British Journal of Clinical Governance*, Vol. 6, No. 2, pp. 129–135.

Naughton, J. (1984) *The Soft Systems Approach: Soft Systems Analysis: An Introductory Guide*, Milton Keynes Open University Press.

West, M. (2002) "The link between the management of employees and patient mortality in acute hospitals", *International Journal of Human Resource Management*, Vol. 13, No. 8, pp 1299–1310.

CHAPTER NINETEEN

The problem with dissecting a frog (is that when you are finished it doesn't really look like a frog anymore)

Andrew Scowcroft

A clash of learning cultures

The first time I found myself explaining Action Learning sets to a group of clinicians (predominantly doctors), I was a worried man. The setting was a management development programme designed by an NHS Trust for its senior consultants, during which there was a slot for someone to come and explain the Action Learning approach, so that participants could decide whether to engage in the process both during and after their formal programme.

I was predicting a clash of learning cultures based on the following stereotypical (but somewhat comfortable) theory. Doctors became doctors by going to lectures, recognising the (temporary) pre-eminence of the lecturer in front of them, writing notes, committing these to memory, and then passing verbal, written and practical exams. Here I was about to articulate something totally contrary to that theory. There was to be no single expert, no uni-directional transfer of knowledge, and no right answer – just lots of talking followed by some doing, and then some more talking! I survived, not due to my oratory or persuasive skills, but through the curiosity and willingness of those same clinicians to 'have a go' – to recognise that there were other ways of learning and problem-solving, and because they could say "NO" at any time!

Of course the original theory was flawed. Clinicians have always learned through conversation with, and critical reflection of, peers and other clinical colleagues. Interestingly, I have found that most of the resistance to the concept and practice of Action Learning has been over the label *"Action Learning"*, and a perception that existing learning techniques and group processes are being given extra and undeserved kudos by association with the latest buzz phrase or label. A common theme in my discussions with medical staff is their perception that management is littered with initiatives and theories that, even if the underlying concept is accepted, suffer from self-aggrandising labels. The purpose of this chapter is not to explore the wider issues of how one profession sees the nomenclature and customs of another, but I raise the issue here because of one stark finding. I have found it much easier to engage clinicians (and it has to be said many other staff groups) if the label Action Learning is downplayed and the discussion focuses directly on the practice and how to get started. The more underpinning theory that is introduced, the more argument and scepticism is generated.

As a direct consequence of that finding, this chapter will not be looking in depth at the background to, or the theories of, Action Learning. It will look instead at a number of practical experiences of the approach, and flag up some of the pitfalls as well as some of the more successful experiences. It will draw extensively upon the author's work in designing, and tutoring on, development programmes, as well as facilitating Action Learning sets for both appointed and elected health leaders.

What we mean

Reginald Revans first articulated Action Learning around fifty years ago (Revans, 1980). Therefore the passage of time, as well as the recent growth in its popularity and use, means that there will be many variations in its implementation. Indeed, a quick search on the Internet will produce a plethora of articles, commercial propositions, and definitions relating to the subject. Revans himself felt that a definition was difficult to provide as the concept was so simple. Definitions I have collected over the years include:

> "A continuous process of learning and reflection, supported by colleagues, with the intention of getting things done."
>
> McGill & Beaty, 1995

and

> "A process that brings people together to find solutions to problems and, in doing so, develops both the individuals and the organisation."
>
> Inglis, 1994

There are many more, but the common theme is that Action Learning can be defined as a process in which a group of people come together more or less regularly to help each other to learn from and then act upon, their experience. Revans coined the phrase "comrades in adversity" to reinforce the need for those involved in the process to have real purpose and commitment to the process, and for all to be able to assist in finding, and then using, new solutions to problems. His vision, backed up by the work he had done at Cambridge University, in the coal industry and with the NHS in the UK, and his latter experiences in Europe, was that the people with the problem should be given the time and space to solve their common problems, through discussion, challenge and implementation. Mineshaft supervisors and ward sisters were, he felt, better placed to both understand and tackle their respective issues than their higher managers.

On the one occasion I met Reginald Revans he was as passionate about Action Learning as he was scathing about management consultants. This was not because of the latter's ability or lack thereof, but because they could not possibly share the "adversity" of those at the coal-face, and therefore their solutions were likely to be abstract and impersonal. He also suggested, somewhat unfairly I thought, that consultancy was all about offering solutions for money, not for learning. I know what he meant but it seemed to tar everyone with the same brush.

The link between Action Learning and leadership development

Readers new to the Action-Learning label may now feel that it is primarily a problem-solving tool. If so, the connection with leadership development seems tenuous at best. How can something designed to help people with problems tackle them differently – a process which seems quite properly rooted in operational management territory – have a place in the development of today's and tomorrows leaders? The answer, as with most things, is in how it is used.

Other chapters of this book explore both the characteristics and behaviours of leaders and the art and practice of leadership. My own view is that, in part, leaders demonstrate leadership by being trusted. Followers in any organisation need to have sufficient faith in their appointed/elected/imposed leaders before they keep their side of the leadership bargain and become fully engaged followers. For me, trust is not just the well-worn concept of having integrity, reliability, and honesty, however important those values are. Being trusted comes from having trusted others first – from having modelled trusting behaviour. Surely leadership involves sometimes saying "I don't know – I really think you might have the better insight" and meaning it, not just testing staff to see if their thinking is as good as yours. Action Learning seems to be a legitimate outcome of leaders asking that question, so it makes sense for developing leaders to have exposure to the approach. This way they will see, and have greater confidence in, the results of their leadership behaviour.

This approach is also consistent with Hersey and Blanchard's work on situational leadership (1988), where they argue that the leader's behaviour ought to be guided by the level of development need of the follower rather than any predetermined leadership style. In particular their work suggests that followers who have demonstrated both ability and self-motivation require a leadership approach based on trust and delegation. Fledgling leaders who have a default style of telling and directing may need to experience what happens when other leaders let go and trust their staff to solve their own problems. Adair, on the front cover of his book "Not Bosses But Leaders" (Adair and Reed, 1987) asserts that

> "You can be appointed a manager, but you are not appointed leader until your appointment is ratified in the hearts and minds of those who work with you".

Another argument for claiming that Action Learning is, or could be, a leadership development tool is that it promotes the collaborative approach to complex issues that leaders in both public and private industry are being encouraged to embrace. The NHS's current concentration on health economies, joint health and local government initiatives, and the general political encouragement to engage in joined-up working, all point to collaboration as the preferred model of organisational leadership behaviour. Action Learning seems highly congruent with joined-up working. Firstly, it looks for shared exploration of new approaches, as opposed to selling existing solutions to the others in the set. Secondly, it promotes the harnessing of all perspectives, building on both insights and experiences. Thirdly, through its name, it places an emphasis on doing something with the learning –on making a difference, from which further learning can occur. Finally it celebrates "we", not "me" or "us and them".

My work with Local Health Boards, NHS Trusts, and devolved Government agencies continues to confirm that an old-style, conveyor-belt, approach to health management whereby each agency does a care-fully-defined task in the supply chain before handing it over to the next link, works against the pursuit of genuine and lasting change. For example, many health practitioners and commentators saw the advent of the commissioner/provider split introduced in the early 1990s (once it was uncoupled from the divisive contract culture) as a useful distinction. It clarified who did what, reduced duplication and conflicts of interest, and sharpened accountability. Quite true and highly desirable. However it was based on a significant but fragile premise – that only those with responsibility for commissioning could "solve" commissioning problems and ditto for provider problems. It failed to acknowledge the fact that providers made commissioning plans work (or not), and that commissioners saw provider activity from a different, and potentially useful, perspective. In the intervening years representatives of both types of health organisation have continued to share problems but *despite* the structure, rather than within the structure. Action Learning seems admirably suited to bringing the various agencies together in a new spirit of collaborative learning, as it provides a legitimate forum for truly collaborative leadership activity to flourish.

However, it will not flourish if its practitioners see it merely as a process whereby one party is bullied into easing the problems of another, or even to understand its impact on another. Alas, I have been invited to facilitate too many of these so-called collaborative sessions, where the ill-concealed agenda is to try to bring the other party(ies) "to their senses". One client made it clear to me that the purpose of the newly-formed joint planning forum was to get party X to see the errors of their ways. Once the niceties of the session were out of the way, the discussion quickly fell into a well-entrenched pattern of claim and counterclaim. Both parties looked back on the session and evaluated it on how far the other party had moved, and

I was left wondering how an Action Learning approach might have produced a different climate, one where the issue had joint ownership, where all views were equally valid, and where the solution was of common interest to all.

I feel that the above perspectives, together with other chapters that touch upon Action Learning, do make the case for including Action Learning as a legitimate leadership development activity, without compromising its equally valuable role as a tool for addressing pressing problems. However, some of the ways in which it can be introduced and used may work against that legitimacy. Some of the less helpful approaches can be categorised as

- Sheep-dipping
- Over-dissection
- A triumph of process over purpose.

Sheep-dipping

I have witnessed a genuinely intended, but potentially damaging, drift towards "Action Learning with everything", whereby programmes are offered with Action Learning as an integral, non-negotiable, ingredient. In this way sheep are dipped in the same solution, regardless of their specific and unique set of needs. I have less concern over those programme providers that include the subject in order to explain it, and then work with those who wish to take it further, but I have witnessed the rather messy aftermath of learning sets that were a compulsory part of the learning experience. One such learning set conspired to meet as expected but then did anything but Action Learning when they were together, preferring to use the time for purely social and/or self indulgent activities. Apart from wasting everyone's time, the experience did little other than confirm a statement made by Rosabeth Moss Kanter at a conference some years ago, that "Powerlessness can corrupt just as easily as can power itself." She argued that if people feel disempowered, they tend to find clandestine ways of "beating the system". In other ways they act in a corrupt way, even if their motives are genuine and human. I know of a case where some office managers who were told that a £50 limit per purchasing order was to be imposed as a way of reducing costs. A legitimate company decision, but imposed rather than developed in conjunction with those who would have to make it work. The managers' response was to contact the supplier and agree that, for big orders, they would be broken down into acceptable sizes, and the invoices would come back to them in £50 chunks. With the system beaten, expenditure went up!

Other learning sets forced to meet, and/or made up of externally-chosen members, have tended to struggle to meet, as the priorities of individuals' own work are genuinely seen as more worthy uses of the time than the learning set meeting. The third undesirable outcome of enforced Action Learning is the tendency to reduce the subject matter to the lowest common denominator. The set slips into a process of finding something, anything, that might be of common interest, rather than assisting one member with a complex issue and seeing how this approach to problems might help them with *their* particular issue. It is this outcome that leads me to caution against too literal an interpretation of Revan's assertion that the problems should be common to all members.

Throughout my careers in both healthcare management and consultancy, there have been times when the significant insight and breakthrough has come from someone who has not shared my problem in the same way as myself. Indeed, if they had, they may have been just as unable as I was to see the wood for the trees. What those individuals did have at the time was a genuine commitment to work with me and to use our discussions to help each other in our work. Many clinicians with whom I have worked in Action Learning sets have commented on how exploring Fred's problem with Bill has helped them with their problem with Jean. They did not both have to deal with Bill, nor did Bill's behaviour have to be the same as Jean's. The common area was more abstract – *dealing with difficult people* – not how to deal with a specific situation. I find some Action Learning sets seek in vain for the ideal problem, one where all members can feel the same pain, when all that is needed is an acceptance that the principles could apply to all. It is this legalistic "painting by numbers" approach to Action Learning that can come from its imposition, however genuine the reasons for such action.

Action Learning is by definition learner-centred. My other worry about "Action Learning with everything" is that it places the organiser's agenda first. It does not signify trust that the action learners, in engaging with the process, will help solve organisational problems. It says that *we* the organisation have problems, and *you* the action learners will come together to solve them. My most worrying example of this was several years ago where an organisation that had engaged fully with the Total Quality Management (TQM) movement, and had set up Quality Improvement Groups (QIGs). This was fine and everyone knew the rationale for those. However when the inevitable dip in concentration came, and the process was seen to be in need of a face-lift, the name was changed to Action Learning. One ex-QIG member said to me, when I was introducing Action Learning on a subsequent multi-professional management development programme, "Oh yes, that's where the organisation gets the staff to solve the managers' problems for them". Their comments were inaccurate (even if genuinely felt) but the effect on the fellow-participants was to place Action Learning firmly at the bottom of their list of legitimate learning methods. Subsequent conversations with the individual revealed that their animosity came from two sources. First was management's insistence that Action Learning was to be an institutionalised part of quality improvement, and secondly, that the topics to be addressed were only influenced at the margins by the set members themselves. Of course this can be dismissed as one person's bad experience, but for me it does point out how any form of imposition can undermine the learning experience, and produce the opposite of the desired result. If people do not learn they do not change. If people are told to learn they will not. If people are invited to learn, they may, and if they choose to learn they will. "What's in it for me?" may appear to be a rather grubby, self-serving question, but it drives much of what we choose to do and adult learning is no different.

Over-dissection

Biology was not my strong point at school. I may have done some form of dissection but I have no memories of it and have to rely on vicarious experience via my daughters' accounts of the process. However a telling phrase enters my mind whenever the subject is mentioned – *"the more you dissect a frog, the less it looks like a frog"*. Whilst I believe that much should be researched and written about important subjects such as Action Learning, (hence this chapter!) I see a real danger in over-explaining it, as there is no real substitute for getting stuck in and doing it (your way).

This brings me to a regular occurrence when I am asked to explain Action Learning to medical staff as part of clinical leadership programmes. The audiences have tended to split into two distinct camps. There are those who want to know the theory, hear of and test the evidence that it works, be given a structure/process, and thus discover "the proper way". The second group find that the more analysis and discussion that takes place, the less attractive the whole thing becomes. During such sessions there is an audible sigh of relief by the latter when the whole group is given an opportunity to try it out, although the first group still seem to want to rely on the "running order" they have winkled out of me earlier. As someone who still naively wants to leave a group having met all of their needs, these sessions leave me, and I suspect, some of the participants, dissatisfied; knowing less about the essence of the "frog" because its rather tangled remains are scattered across the table.

I am increasingly finding myself wanting to tackle the introduction of Action Learning by engaging in Action Learning, rather then spend a long time talking about it first. This approach still allows the theoretical and analytical dimension to be explored, but *in* the here-and-now of experiencing the environment of Action Learning.

As an example, at the time of writing I am working with one NHS client where the need is for a short, focused, practical skills-based programme for new clinical directors. The group is mainly, but not exclusively, made up of doctors. What we have devised is an approach where, during each of seven half day sessions, the first hour will be more of a technical presentation by a local "expert" on issues related to strategic and operational management; understanding the local financial arrangements and how to bid for service improvement funding; managing medical politics; leading multi professional teams, etc. The reminder of the time has been labelled "Surgery" where the nine participants can bring topical issues connected to, and stimulated by, the theme of the session and build on each others' insight and experiences. The modular approach will allow time for some degree of implementation and experimentation of any new approaches, before they meet again as well as allowing the participants to *own the process* and *stop/change it at any time*. Notice that there is no mention of the Action Learning label and no big launch. The whole initiative is based on finding out what it is that these people need now to do the management/leadership aspects of their new jobs and then creating conditions where those needs can be met. Therefore the initiative meets the "What's in it for me?" litmus test, and honours the twin principles of Action Learning – learning and doing.

In part the approach has its genealogy in a comment from John Harvey Jones' book "Making It Happen" (Harvey Jones, 1988), where he points out that:

> "In my experience it is impossible to teach grown up people anything. However it is possible to create conditions where they will teach themselves."

Triumph of process over purpose

Practitioners of the Myers Briggs Type Indicator or MBTI (Briggs Myers *et al.*, 1998) will be well aware of the differences in psychological type among people, and that some prefer structure whilst others respond more comfortably to freedom and ambiguity. I regularly use these concepts to help teams and groups become more effective, by accepting that differences can be healthy rather than irritating, and that they can be used properly rather than denied or changed. The key is to use all perspectives, matched to the needs of the team at that time, and not to favour one approach as a matter of team policy. Action Learning requires that same balanced approach. It requires sufficient process to make relevant use of the time and resources of the set, coupled with space to be "beside the point" and an early warning system for the set becoming victims of their own process.

Mention the hilarious training film "Meetings Bloody Meetings", and many a manager's eyes will water. They will recall the incompetent chairing skills of John Cleese's character; the meetings with no purpose and outcome; the sheer uselessness and repetitiveness of the agenda, and the complete disillusionment of the other team members. Clinical readers of this book may not have seen this seminal video but your local training department is still likely to have a copy. Most viewers find it worryingly easy to compare some of its scenarios with their own experiences, and many shuffle uncomfortably in their seats whist watching the film. Why then do so many NHS meeting attendees, be they for clinical, strategy, planning, Action Learning or other reasons, go to each one with a sense of doom and come away with a vow never to attend again?

Whilst Action Learning should never be viewed as the same sort of meeting as, say, a management board, or a medical staff committee, there are a few common principles. These are:

1. The need for clarity of purpose, both in terms of the overall reason for the people to be together, and for each specific session
2. The need for sufficient process to guide the participants to their agreed destination
3. The need for that forum to do only that which it is best placed to do, and not attempt to do what is best done elsewhere, and
4. The explicit ownership of the way in which the group works, so that it can change when it needs to, and not wait to be changed from the outside.

In my experience Action Learning, (whether called this or not) that has worked as a clinical leadership tool, has recognised these four principles and the action learners have taken it upon themselves to establish a balance that works for them. Where and when the process overwhelms or becomes a substitute for purpose, items three and four in the above list become a problem.

One clinically-based Action Learning set that I worked with in its latter stages had designed an impressive process. The structure of sessions contained minute-by-minute timings; the responsibility for room and domestic arrangements was democratically shared out; the dates were set six months in advance; the desirable topics brainstormed and scheduled into the various meetings and the "facilitator" role was rotated amongst the set. Its early meetings were reported by the set members as useful, productive, focused and "successful". There were disagreements and tensions but nothing that highly qualified clinicians did not deal with on a daily basis back at work.

One particular session tackled "how to influence the strategic direction of the service, without being seen as shroud wavers" (their description, not mine). The session itself went well by all accounts, but the topic was so fundamental to the work of many of the set members that it needed more time. It should have led to a discussion about, temporarily, putting on hold the set programme and working the issues through, potentially for a few more sessions. Some members wanted to, others felt that they would never get onto the other topics if one topic dominated the discussion. From that point on the eight members of the learning set effectively divided into two sub-sets, each of which pursued their different preferred discussion in the same room. The following session began to tackle the next subject on the list, but soon the discussion drifted, or was pulled, back to the previous issue. The nominated "facilitator" felt pulled two ways, and was damned whichever option he or she suggested. Towards the end of this phase, the set members began to abandon both the hot topic of influencing the strategic agenda, and the scheduled topic of the day, and used the time to prepare for, or grumble about, other work meetings they had attended, engaging in what several set members admitted was gossip about colleagues. Attendance began to wane as the atmosphere, as well as the outcomes of the time spent, began to compare very unfavourably with the alternative uses of the time back at work, and those who came exuded resentment that this session was happening by arriving late and leaving early. By the time I was approached, by one of the learning set members, the set was experiencing death by apathy.

All four of those earlier principles were at work here, but pulling in different directions.

Firstly, there had been some attempt to articulate purpose at the outset, but it was fairly superficial, and related to a general intention to discuss "the issues we all face as clinicians". This was accurate but did not go far enough. It did not allow any degree of priority or assessment of critical issues as compared to "life's ups and downs". It seemed not to capture the heart of Action Learning which is to jointly seek new approaches and try them out, with the result that many of the discussions involved one person suggesting/telling the others what they should do, on the basis that they had already been there and done that. The contradiction between the expectation of "collaborative discussion" and the reality of "expert advice sessions" was never explicitly challenged. The triumph of one over the other led to the sessions becoming very similar to a grand round, or a topic tutorial.

Secondly, with the lack of depth to the purpose of the set, the initial process of brainstorming issues simply reinforced each topic as having equal status, equal hurt, equal complexity, and therefore an assumption that it could be dealt with in an equal amount of time. "If it's October, it must be budgets!" became the inevitable consequence of planning content so far ahead. The process was efficient, discharged professionally and democratically, yet moved further and further away from meeting the needs of the set.

Thirdly, rather than tackle directly the symptoms and causes of their difficulty, the set members tacitly conspired to simply change the nature of their discussion onto new common ground. Turning the sessions into talking shops for their minor grumbles about their place of work is something that they might have criticised others for doing, but were initially unaware they were sliding into the same trap. The set stopped doing those things it was uniquely equipped to do, and started to be seen as yet another unproductive use of time.

Fourthly, because the scene setting and purpose work was so thin, no one seemed able or supported enough to bring the process to a halt and say "Let's review and rethink this approach, and decide whether we need to agree a new purpose/process." It was almost as if the set felt that someone one else had imposed the format and they were unable to change it. Returning to the potential of powerlessness to corrupt, the set members were making the set fail rather than discussing how to make it work in the light of a new situation. One set member suggested at the time that Action Learning was akin to the emperors new clothes – beautifully explained and promoted, but ultimately transparent and devoid of content. Ironically he was one of the original champions of the highly-detailed process

My involvement focused initially on making *how* the set worked as important a discussion topic as the original content they had devised. Whilst this might sound somewhat artificial out of context, the set was encouraged to spend some time at each session critiquing the session itself and, if necessary, proposing changes for next time. The set became more adaptable and dynamic as a result and process became a tool of the set rather than a straightjacket for the set to wear.

We also strengthened the overall purpose of the group so that it emphasised critical issues and the need to effect changes, to learn by doing. This, together with the increased ownership, allowed the set to identify a much more robust and relevant shortlist of issues and an agreement to devote the time needed to each as opposed to working through a timetable. The new preparedness to take stock at regular intervals not only improved the problem solving process for each issue, it provided the clues to when it was time to move on. In this way those with a preference for structure and order had their needs met, and those who needed the freedom to stay with an issue were similarly satisfied.

The final demonstration of ownership was that, without any rancour or grand gestures, three members of the set decided that their needs would be best met in other ways and they withdrew, wishing the set well in its endeavours.

Beyond the particular environments of learning sets, I continue to see examples of process triumphing over purpose and outcome. Teams that have meetings on a Wednesday, because it is the 'Wednesday Meeting', where the only change to the content and layout of the agenda is the date at the top, where viewing the meeting's entry in the diary makes the heart sink and where participants view themselves as more victims of the process than owners and designers. In the hurly burly of organisational life, there is only so much that can be changed by one person, but Action Learning ought to be a beacon of light for ownership, the courage to change, accepting personal responsibility for good and bad experiences and creating the right environment. In other words, a place where leaders can learn many of the components of good leadership

Overall my experiences have led me to conclude that there are four key determinants of Action Learning as a positive leadership development tool. These are, in no particular order of priority,

- The contexts in which it is introduced and used,
- Its congruence with the cultural environment of the organisations in which its participants operate,
- The mindset of its participants, and
- Its ongoing management/facilitation.

These themes provide some loose structure for the conclusion of this chapter, although the links between the five may lead to some blurring of the edges at times.

The contexts

In my work as an independent management development consultant, NHS organisations have asked me to design and run large-scale management and leadership development programmes, and/or contribute to Action Learning initiatives, mostly in the form of external facilitation of learning sets. From these experiences, I detect three main contexts for Action Learning:

1. Action Learning as a planned, timetabled activity interwoven with the other formal aspects of a programme, with the Action Learning set either ceasing at the end of the programme or being allowed/encouraged to continue in a self managed way for as long as set members derive benefit,

2. Action Learning as an activity introduced towards the end of a formal programme, with the organiser's anticipation that some participants would form an Action Learning set as a way of continuing their development, bridging the potential divide between the programme and work,

3. Action Learning as a discrete leadership development activity in its own right, neither relying on nor continuing the momentum of, a formal programme.

I have experienced more of the first two than the third, and it is interesting to explore why that might be.

On the positive side, it makes sense for providers of management and leadership development to allow, or even, encourage, participants to explore a wide range of learning methods. Whether using the Learning Styles Questionnaire (Honey & Mumford, 1986), itself based on Kolb's learning cycle (1984), or reflecting on personality preferences as explored by instruments such as the MBTI, there is an increasing recognition that we operate and therefore learn in different ways. Some seem to benefit more from critical exploration of a topic, in the here and now of dealing with it, whereas others may extract more long-term learning from observing "from a distance", and so on. As with most experiences in life, there is an element of "you don't know what you don't know", and it could be argued that, without some enforced exposure to something like Action Learning via a development programme, few would embrace unstructured group learning alongside other job pressures. In discussion with colleagues and clients, it appears more common for NHS staff to have their first exposure to Action Learning as part of a formal programme and, in my experience, almost all medical staff fall into this category.

On the negative side, there are risks that the initiative could be seen as evidence of the sheep-dipping approach discussed earlier, or meeting the provider's philosophy of what constitutes learning. In my experience, such views come from perceptions rather than the explicit aims of development programme providers, but a person's perception is that person's reality and should be carefully considered.

For me the key redeeming feature of the first two contexts is that there is (eventually, in the first example) an explicit transfer of ownership and choice. Once the formal programme is concluded, the existence, content, style, and outcomes of any Action Learning approach are all in the hands of those who wish to engage. I believe that any attempt by the organisers to impose Action Learning after a formal programme, even if it is able to retain willing learning set members, is meeting its own agenda rather than that of the set members and does Action Learning a disservice.

Other benefits of the third context are that the coming together of people is more natural, and spontaneous; that the issues are likely to drive the need for Action Learning and the make-up of any particular set, and that ownership is there from the start, so it does not need to be handed over. Conversely, the main risk is that it will never happen at all. Whatever my personal wishes about more people being able to experience and them come to an informed view about Action Learning, I do not see it spontaneously breaking out in the manner of a Welsh Valleys religious Revival! This brings me to the real double-edged sword of Action Learning as a leadership development tool. At the risk of mixing my metaphors, it needs the oxygen of publicity and some competent explanation, for the seeds to be planted, yet at the same time it loses some if its essence when part of a organised initiative, or when accompanied by great form and ceremony. For me the secret of avoiding cuts from the double-edged sword lies in the culture of organisations.

Culture

This chapter does not seek to describe or analyse organisational culture, nor does it provide labels. However, I do see some basic cultural ingredients that have to be in place if Action Learning is to have a proper place on the leadership development map.

Firstly, the organisation needs to be prepared to accept learning and insight wherever it emerges, and have robust internal mechanisms for celebrating both success and "nice tries". I frequently listen to project-related presentations given by participants of both Action Learning sets and formal development programmes. A recurring thought is – how could others in this organisation hear of this work so that they do not reinvent either the wheel or the flat tyre?

Some professions have developed forums for discussing issues of common concern (e.g., Trust professional nurse forums) but they seem underused as places for one team's learning to be celebrated, and the medical profession in particular has no obvious equivalent. I would go further and suggest that some senior executives of health organisations seem genuinely surprised when they see or hear of more junior staff succeeding at something "difficult". In such circumstances the staff member's pride at being recognised is all but cancelled out by the impression that their higher leaders did not think they could do it!

When Action Learning is undertaken by people from different organisations (cultures), a new set of challenges emerges. For example, how does a learning set (the collective name given to a group of action learners) cope when some return to an organisation whose staff are encouraged to experiment, reflect, and develop, while others find that their learning set commitment is simply viewed by colleagues and bosses as avoiding the "real" work? One of the common reasons for Action Learning sets failing or for individual members withdrawing, is increasing frustration at being unable to experiment. It seems self-evident that an organisational culture that encourages and rewards joined-up thinking; acknowledges that complex problems require time and space and is genuinely willing to learn as much from nice tries as from clear successes without instilling fear into staff, is likely to provide fertile ground for collaborative learning. That is not to say that Action Learning cannot be found in less supportive cultures, simply that in such situations the process, and its participants, are more likely to be viewed with suspicion or indifference. I have observed both types of culture, and a third that is probably more challenging. This is the environment where risk, experimentation and support are preached, but the consequences of failure are career limiting. The need for an explicit link between Action Learning and leadership development is critically important in such cultures.

The mindset of its participants

A common routine for new action learners to fall into is that of selling solutions to their colleagues. Most senior managers and clinicians enter the Action Learning environment from a place where quick decision-making is the norm, where more junior colleagues come for advice and direction, and where the rewarded behaviour is making problems "go away". It can be quite difficult for such individuals to slow down and work collaboratively, even if they have joined an Action Learning set specifically to "get away from the day-to-day rush". My work with clini-cally-based Action Learning sets suggest that, as a profession, medicine is particularly prone to this quick-fire, telling and selling approach. Recent work with one particular learning set involved hearing several statements preceded by "Well – what you need to do about that is…." It is interest-ing to note that both giver and receiver of this advice found benefit from the experience, but I detected that the others in the room were reduced to the role of spectator. In my opinion it is vital that, even if a set mem-ber offers a solution, the whole set is willing and able to hold that idea and develop it further, rather than simply watch something that worked in one cultural environment being forced upon another culture. In other words the mindset of the group has to be to find new approaches – after all if the existing approaches all worked, there would be no need for the set in the first place. This mindset of holding issues and spending time exploring why it may or may not work, is the significant difference between Action Learning and the other labels mentioned above. F. Scott Fitzgerald rather encouragingly suggested that

> "The test of a first rate intelligence is the ability to hold two opposed ideas in the mind at the same time, and still retain the ability to function."
>
> Scott Fitzgerald, 1936

This involves slowing down, nurturing those different ideas rather than trying to kill one of them. In short, it requires the set to be comfortable with uncertainty and ambiguity. This can be unfamiliar territory for many clinicians and managers especially if they see their role as the pursuit of solutions (i.e., certainty). This change of approach may take time to develop and some sets look for some facilitative guidance at the start.

Ongoing management/facilitation

As someone who makes part of his living from facilitation, I need to tread the fine line between objective conclusions from my experience and appearing to promote my services. Therefore let me say at once that the best Action Learning sets are the ones that run themselves, for there lies ownership, responsibility to change purpose and process, and the bravery to stop when the set no longer meets the members' needs. However, given that Action Learning for some is a significant step away from their normal work environment, it makes sense for the early period to be supported by gentle advice and facilitation, although this should be offered rather than imposed.

Calculators out! Action Learning is not cheap. If a set comprising of, say, six medical consultants, engage in six two-hour sessions the overall time with travel will easily exceed 72 hours at the current hourly rate, so the economic risks of going off in the wrong direction still need to be managed. If asked to work with a set, I usually ask them two questions. The first is what they want from me and the second is when do they think they will not need me. Sets usually ask for help in keeping them focused, preventing time-wasting, and an objective perspective – just what I would have offered but it was better for them to think it through and to ask first. Sets are less clear about the second question but, having asked it up front, I am able to return to it naturally as the set matures, rather than appear to be losing interest or wanting to abandon the set. Many sets start, develop, and disband perfectly well with out any external assistance, and others merely need a local guide to provide "telephone" advice. Nevertheless, given all of my earlier comments, it is clear that Action Learning, especially when involving busy clinical staff, can suffer all too easily from not being set up correctly. I am constantly reminded of the old mantra of *form follows function*, and it seems admirably suited for

Action Learning. Once you decide explicitly what it is that you want the set to do, it is much easier to set up processes, timetables, review mechanisms etc, that get you there. The alternative (where function follows form) seems to me a poor return for the twin investment of taxpayers money and scarce clinical time.

Conclusion

I believe that Action Learning should take its place as one of several methods of leadership development. It should not be forced, although it does seem to make sense to raise its profile on formal programmes if only to allow participants to become aware and make an informed decision. It is a technique admirably suited to modelling both leadership behaviour and the new agenda of inter-agency collaborative working. When it works well, it provides new solutions, new thinking and enhanced learning for those involved. When it falters, it normally does so due to enforced application or lack of clarity of its purpose, and both of these conditions can be easily cured.

I conclude with two messages, one for organisations and one for current or future action learners. To organisations I would ask them to seek out and celebrate anything that involves colleagues coming together to explore new approaches, but then leave people to it. Rather like David Attenborough brings to our attention the myriad nature of the world around us, raises its profile, but does not seek to change or occupy it, leaders and staff developers need to be champions of Action Learning, not colonialists. For individuals the message is simple – make it yours. If Action Learning is learning whilst doing, then make the learning yours, and make the doing yours. If you bring to the set problems and issues you face at work, your organisation will benefit from the actions you take just as much as you will benefit from the learning process.

Leadership and management can be lonely businesses, but they don't need to be if you see those around you as fellow learners. Winnie the Pooh was both leader of his particular 'organisation' and an ideal action learner. Here's the evidence!

> "When you are a Bear of Very Little Brain, and you think things, you
> find sometimes that a Thing that was very Thingish inside you is

quite different when it gets out in the open and has other people looking at it."

Milne, 1928

References

Adair, J. & Reed, P. (1987) *Not Bosses but Leaders*, London, Kogan Page.

Briggs Myers. I., McCaulley, M., Quenk, N. & Hammer, A. (1998) *Myers Briggs Type Instrument: Manual*, Palo Alto, Consulting Psychologists Press.

Harvey Jones, J. (1988) *Making it Happen: Reflections on Leadership*, London, Harper Collins.

Hersey, P. & Blanchard, K. (1988) *The Management of Organizational Behavior: Utilising Human Resources*, Englewood Cliffs, Prentice-Hall.

Honey, P. & Mumford, A. (1986) *The Manual of Learning Styles*, Maidenhead, Peter Honey Publications.

Inglis, S. (1994) *Making the Most of Action Learning*, Aldershot, Gower.

Kolb, D. (1984) *Experiential Learning: Experience as the Source of Learning and Development*, Englewood Cliffs, Prentice-Hall.

McGill, I. & Beaty, L (1995) *Action Learning: A Practitioner's Guide,* 2nd edition, London, Kogan Page.

Milne, A. (1928) *The House at Pooh Corner*, London, Methuen.

Revans, R. (1980) *Action Learning: New Techniques for Management,* London, Blond & Briggs.

Scott Fitzgerald, F. (1936) "The crack up", *Esquire Magazine* (February).

Index